STUDIES ON WINES

AND

FUEL ALCOHOL PRODUCTION

Nandita Gupta

जय गुरुदेव

© 2022, Author

ISBN13: 978-93-95766-39-5 Paperback Edition
ISBN13: 978-93-95766-40-1 Hardbound Edition
ISBN13: 978-93-95766-41-8 Digital Edition
This work is licensed under a Creative Commons Attribution 4.0 International License. Please visit
https://creativecommons.org/licenses/by/4.0/

Title: **Studies on Wines and Fuel Alcohol Production**
Author: **Nandita Gupta**

Printed and Published by
Devotees of Sri Sri Ravi Shankar Ashram
34 Sunny Enclave, Devigarh Road,
Patiala 147001, Punjab, India

https://advaita56.in/
The Art of Living Centre

30th May 2022 1:08pm Monday, Sunny Enclave Home Bedroom. Mummy attains param samadhi in the lap of Papa while Ashwini is writing Ashtavakra Gita, Sangeeta is at work, Dipanshu is at Sri Sri University Orissa, Richa has gone for Yoga and Dance.

On this day in 1431 French heroine Jeanne d'Arc (Joan of Arc) attains samadhi, 1606 Guru Arjun Dev attains samadhi, 2000 Shania Twain wins Country Music award, 2012 Vishwanathan Anand wins his 5th World Chess Championship, 2019 Brigitte Bierle is first female chancellor of Austria, 2020 SpaceX Falcon 9 rocket ferries astronauts to Space Station for 1st time.

Vikram Samvat 2079 Nala, Saka Era 1944 Shubhakrit

1st Edition May 2022

जय गुरुदेव

Specially Dedicated to

My beloved Mother KAVITA PAUL AGGARWAL who attained final liberation at home on Monday 30th May 2022 at 1:08pm afternoon peacefully in divine sleep.

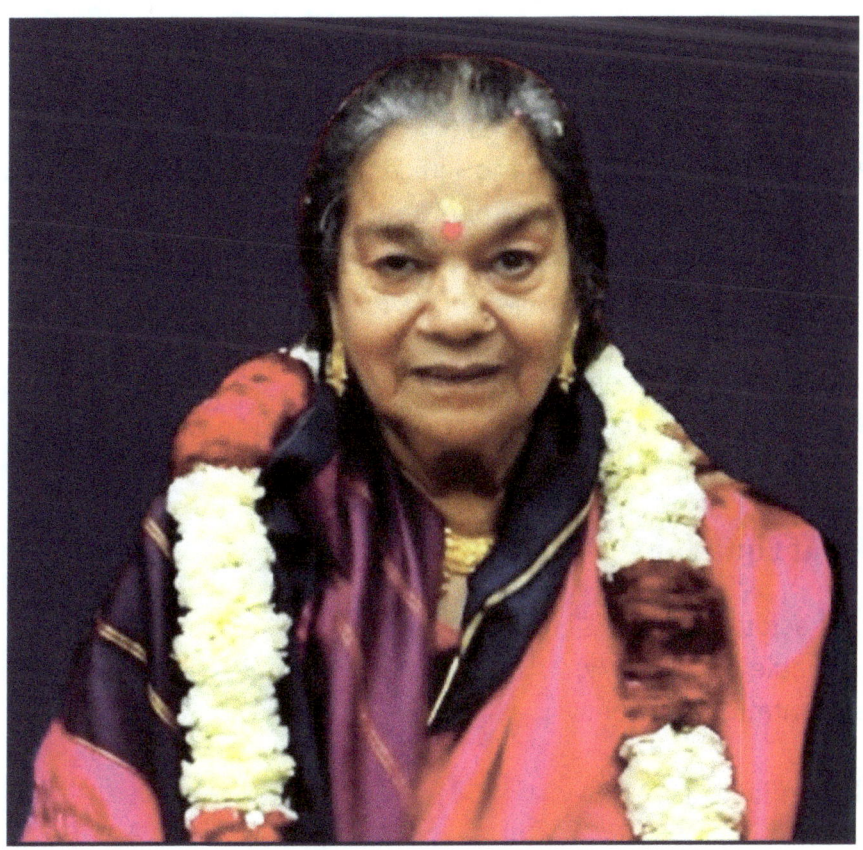

List of Figures

Fig 1: Immature Mango Fruit	24
Fig 2: Discolored Mango Fruit	24
Fig 3: Ruptured Mango Fruit	25
Fig 4: Mango Fruit Damaged by Birds	25

List of Tables

Table 1: Composition of mango juice* (**Var. Dussehri**)	33
Table 2: TSS vs Alcoholic Fermentation	36
Table 3: Inoculum vs Alcoholic Fermentation	38
Table 4: Fermentation Temp. vs Alcoholic Fermentation	41
Table 5: pH vs Alcoholic Fermentation	44
Table 6: KMS vs Alcoholic Fermentation	46
Table 7: Optimum conditions for prod. of mango wine	47
Table 8: Analysis of Mango wine	48

List of Equations

Total acidity (% w/v)	29
% Volatile acidity (w/v)	29
Fermentation efficiency	31

Abbreviations

v/v = volume/volume, w/v = weight in volume
°C = degree Celsius, °B = degree Brix
KMS = Potassium metabisulphite

STUDIES ON WINES AND FUEL ALCOHOL PRODUCTION

BY

NANDITA PAUL
(L-89-BS-100-M)

THESIS

Submitted to the Punjab Agricultural University
in partial fulfillment of the requirements
for the degree of

MASTER OF SCIENCE
IN
MICROBIOLOGY

[Minor Field: Food Science & Technology]

Department of Microbiology
College of Basic Science & Humanities
PUNJAB AGRICULTURAL UNIVERSITY
LUDHIANA - 141004

1991

DEDICATED TO

MY RESPECTED

PARENTS

CERTIFICATE I

This is to certify that this thesis entitled "Studies on Wines and Fuel Alcohol Production" submitted for the degree of Master of Science in the subject of Microbiology [Minor Field: Food Science and Technology] of the Punjab Agricultural University, is a bonafide research work carried out by Nandita Paul (L-89-BS-100-M) under my supervision and that no part of this thesis has been submitted for any other degree.

The assistance and help received during the course of investigation have been fully acknowledged.

[Dr H. K. Tewari]
Major Advisor
Mycologist
Dept. of Microbiology
Punjab Agricultural University
LUDHIANA

CERTIFICATE II

This is to certify that the thesis entitled "Studies on Wines and Fuel Alcohol Production" submitted by Nandita Paul (L-89-BS-100-M) to the Punjab Agricultural University in partial fulfilment of the requirements for the degree of Master of Science in the subject of Microbiology [Minor field: Food Science and Technology] has been approved by the Student's Advisory Committee after an oral examination on the same, in collaboration with an external examiner.

17.2.1992

Major Advisor   **External Examiner**
(Dr. H. K. Tewari)   (Dr. S. S. Marwaha)
HEAD
Dept. of Biotechnology
Punjabi University
PATIALA

20.2.1992
Head of the Department
(Dr. R. S. Kahlon)

5 MAR 1992
Dean, Post-graduate Studies
(Dr. D. S. Sidhu)

ACKNOWLEDGEMENTS

The culmination of this project work is an important landmark in my academic career. For this achievement my heartfelt thanks go to my major advisor, Dr. H. K. Tewari, Mycologist, Department of Microbiology, Punjab Agricultural University, Ludhiana, without whose unflinching support, affectionate and inspiring encouragement, constructive guidance, sound advice and valuable suggestions, this would have been just a dream. This dissertation contains just a fraction of what my great teacher has taught me and has contributed towards the overall development of my personality, enabling me to acquire sufficient moral strength and knowledge to face the various odds of life.

I am profoundly grateful to Dr. P. K. Khanna, Mycologist, Department of Microbiology, for his helpful attitude and valuable suggestions during this study. I also owe my thanks to the other members of my advisory committee, Dr. Ajit Singh, Sr. Microbiologist, Department of Microbiology and Dr. J. S. Kanwar, Professor, Department of Horticultural, for their sincere help and cooperation during the course of this investigation.

I am highly obliged to Dr R. K. Sedha and Dr. Neelam of the Department of Microbiology for allowing me to use the equipment in their laboratory.

It gives me immense pleasure to extend my warmest thanks to all my friends (89 gang) for their affectionate encouragement, enthusiasm and cheerful company. My special thanks are due to Surinder, Rupinder, Alka, Maninder, Anita and Jaswinder.

I am at a loss for words to express my deep sense of gratitude for my respected parents for their hearty blessings and ever encouraging moral support. I am also indebted to my loving brother, Ashwini and sister, Sangeeta, who have always stood by me and been a source of my strength.

Financial assistance in the form of merit fellowship given by Punjab Agricultural University, Ludhiana, during the tenure of my M.Sc. is gratefully acknowledged.

Dated: 30.12.1991   Nandita Paul

Title of Thesis	**Studies on Wines and Fuel Alcohol Production**
Name of Student	Nandita Paul
Admission No.	L-89-BS-100-M
Major Advisor	Dr. H. K. Tewari
Major Subject	Microbiology
Minor Subject	Food Science and Technology
Degree to be awarded	**Master of Science**
Year of award of degree	**1992**
Total pages in thesis	50 + xv
Name of University	**Punjab Agricultural University**, Ludhiana - 141004, India

ABSTRACT

Substandard and waste mango (*Mangifera indica*) var. Dussehri was utilized for ethanol fermentation by *Saccharomyces cerevisiae* var. ellipsoideus strain Montrachet (@ 15% v/v). Ethanol 9.0% v/v was produced from the substrate with initial TSS of 20.0 °B (pH 5.0). The optimum fermentation period was 96 hours at 30 °C. Potassium metabisulphite (KMS @ 50 ppm) prevented contamination. Chemical analysis and sensory evaluation have classified the mango wine as of commercially outstanding quality. Aqueous ethanol was dehydrated with Calcium chloride (@18 gm/100 ml) yielding 99.5% ethyl alcohol which can be used as liquid fuel.

Dr. H. K. Tewari   **Nandita Paul**

Contents

CHAPTER I – INTRODUCTION 1-3

TECHNICAL PROGRAM OF RESEARCH WORK 3

CHAPTER II – REVIEW OF LITERATURE 4-22

I. Ethanol as a Fuel 5
II. Various Substrates for Ethanol Production 6
III. Factors influencing fermentation 10
IV. Production of wines 17
V. Dehydration of Ethanol for fuel 19
VI. Immobilization of Yeasts 20

CHAPTER III – MATERIALS AND METHODS 23-32

CHAPTER IV – RESULTS AND DISCUSSION 33-48

CHAPTER V - SUMMARY 49-50

LITERATURE CITED .... I-XV

APPENDIX I I

PUBLISHER'S ADDENDUM .... A

Scans of Original (some) .... A
Acknowledgements (part portion) .... B
References .... D

EPILOGUE .... F

Chapter I – INTRODUCTION

The application of improved agricultural practices and development of new fruit varieties has led to an increase in the fruit production in the country during the last decade. India is one of the largest producers of fruits and vegetables in the world with an annual production of about 70 million tons. Less than two lakh tons of fruits and vegetables are utilized for processing and preservation, Approximately 15 million tons of horticultural produce, equivalent of its market cost of Rs 3,000 crores, goes down the drain every year in our country. This is because efforts have not been directed seriously to control the fruit and vegetable wastage. In Punjab state 25-30% of fruits and 15-40% of vegetables are wasted. The fruit production in this state is likely to be doubled by 1995 as per the estimates of the Johl's Committee on the Diversification of Agriculture.

The recent increase in the anticipated improvement in the fruit production in the coming years have created post-harvest problems for the progressive fruit growers in the country and the Punjab in particular. Mango is the first most important fruit of Punjab state. It is grown on 26,340 acres producing 65,850 tons of fruits annually. The Dussehri variety of Mango ripens in late June and during this season it becomes practically inconvenient for the fruit growers to store the harvest at a very high temperature (40 ±2 °C or above). They have to store their produce in cold storages for sale during the off-season or transport to other places or dispose off the produce at throw-away prices in the local market. Though the cold storages have played a significant role in the preservation of fruits but this facility is inadequate to meet the requirements of the farmers. Transportation and improper handling also result in substandard fruits. Good quality fruits are accepted for table purposes whereas discolored, injured, immature and bird-eaten fruits (Figure 1-4) have no commercial value. Such fruits are either sold at a very low price or disposed off, on land in open, resulting in environmental pollution. All these practices mean incurring additional capital and consequently economic losses to the progressive fruit growers.

Although horticulture has ushered in an economic boom in Punjab state, yet it has not so far received adequate attention to process substandard or waste fruits. In the absence of this, the farmers continue to have unremunerative prices. The processing of surplus fruits into commercially acceptable products like juice, jams, jelly, etc. seem to be an answer to the post-harvest problems of the fruit growers, but the growth of the fruit processing industries in the country and in Punjab, in particular, is very limited due to some technical and other constraints. The utilization of substandard, low-grade and surplus produce for the production of quality wines and fuel alcohol will improve the economics of the fruit production and control the environmental pollution caused by decaying fruit.

Alcohol production is largely synthetic although the rising costs of petroleum have renewed interest in the production of fuel alcohol by fermentation. Ethanol can be produced from horticultural raw and waste materials containing starch or fermentable sugars. Ethanol is used for multiple purposes in chemical industries. It is in great demand for the manufacture of alcoholic drinks. Ethanol also possesses many characteristics of an ideal fuel. It does not increase amount of carbon dioxide in the atmosphere, thus causes less air pollution. Industrial alcohol has been valuable as a solvent, germicide, antifreeze, fuel and chemical raw material.

Keeping the above facts in view, the present investigation has been undertaken to explore the possibilities for the production of ethanol by fermenting substandard mango. The objectives of the investigations were fulfilled by carrying out the work under the following technical program.

Technical Program of Research Work

1. Collection of samples.

2. Analysis of samples for reducing sugars, fermentation temperature, pH, total soluble solids and total acids.

3. Production of wine from mango.

4. Dehydration of aqueous ethanol for energy.

Chapter II – REVIEW OF LITERATURE

Ethanol has been used for feedstock and fuel since a very long time. Archaeological evidences indicate that alcoholic beverage formation was 1,000 years old (Greenshield, 1975). The Arabs and Romans distilled alcohol (Miller, 1975) and Christian monasteries in Europe distilled it as fuel alcohol. Ethanol is being used as a motor fuel since before 1890. But its low heat value prevented any extensive use of it until the World War I. However, during the period of Pre-World War II, the increasing demand for antiknock fuels and perfection of processes for production of anhydrous alcohol, made its use possible.

The energy consumption in the world is increasing at an alarming rate and the non-renewable sources of energy are getting depleted rapidly. This acute energy problem has caused renewed interest in alternative and renewable sources of energy and fuel.

The literature on the production of ethanol from substandard fruits has been reviewed under the following headings:

I. Ethanol as a fuel
II. Substrates for ethanol production
III. Factors influencing fermentation
IV. Production of wines
V. Dehydration of aqueous ethanol for fuel
VI. Immobilization of yeast

I. Ethanol as a Fuel

The preparation of absolute alcohol was first reported in 1796. Extensive industrial use of ethyl alcohol began in the late 1800s (Maioella, 1985).

Since the early days of the automobile, ethanol and ethanol-gasoline mixtures have been considered for use as a fuel. The abundant and less expensive petroleum supply precluded extensive use of ethanol as fuel, and only in the last few years the general public has become aware of and concerned about the dwindling and increasingly expensive petroleum supplies. Interest in extending gasoline supplies with ethanol-gasoline mixtures has increased greatly (Friend and Shahani, 1981).

The properties of alcohol containing gasoline, used as a fuel was described by Matsumoto and Yamamoto (1973). Ethanol increased the octane number and thermal efficiency but lowered the calorific values of the gasoline. The engine resulted in larger fuel consumption but maximum output of engine was not affected.

Alcohol may be used as such or blended with other liquid fuels. Ingamells and Lindquist (1975) described ethanol gasoline blends which are currently marketed commercially. The use of both methanol and ethanol had been very extensive in Europe during the period of pre-World War II (Stone, 1974). Menrad (1977) reviewed the progress in automobile fuels. In India, Jayaraman (1979) demonstrated a car which can run on 100 percent alcohol. Gupta and Ahluwalia (1980) conducted various vehicle tests to determine the feasibility of using 20-30 percent ethanol.

Extensive studies were conducted on the possible alternative to crude oil and the results showed that alcohol, especially ethanol and methanol are the most prominent alternatives (Menrad and Loeck, 1980). The individual process steps for ethanol production as an automotive fuel from agriculture plantation to the final use are all very well developed and technologically investigated by Faust and Prave (1980). Ethanol production from potato and subsequently dehydrated (99.5% v/v) may be used as a blend with other liquid fuels. (Tewari *et al.*, 1982).

Beavan *et al.*, (1989) conducted comparative performance trials with yeast and *Zymomonas* for fuel alcohol production from corn. Archer and Thompson (1987) conducted studies on energy production through treatment of wastes by micro-organisms. The production of methanol and ethanol from wastes already proceeds on an industrial scale. Saida (1989) has described a process for the preparation of ethanol by fermenting a saccharide in a fermentation liquid containing water, utilizing microorganisms.

II. Various Substrates for Ethanol Production

In India, about 30 million tons of fruits and vegetables are produced and out of this over 20 million tons have been fruits only. But hardly one percent of this is utilized for processing and preservation and about 30-33 percent of the total production is wasted due to spoilage during handling, transportation and lack of cold storage facilities (Baisya, 1980).

There has been considerable interest in the production of alcohol from food processing wastes because of the rising energy costs and the negative cost values of wastes as substrates (Hang *et al.*, 1981). Prouty *et al.*, (1980) have discussed the impact of various raw materials and alternate fermentation methods on process designs for the production of fuel grade ethanol.

Production of ethanol from a) sugarcane, b) whey, c) sugar beet, d) banana, e) apple, f) grape, g) pineapple, h) cassava, i) cactus and j) water hyacinth have also been explored by various scientists in the recent years, for their suitability as substances for the production of ethanol by using various microorganisms.

a) Sugarcane

Hartley and Sharma (1987) have reviewed novel ethanol fermentation from sugarcane and straw by a mutant strain of *Bacillus stearothermophilus* at rates equivalent to yeasts.

Thorsson (1989) has described a process for the production of ethanol through molasses fermentation. Ethanol production from sugarcane syrup using *Zymomonas mobilis* has been studied by Doelle and Doelle (1989). Novel supplements like skim milk, chitin and fungal mycelium, enhance the ethanol production in cane molasses fermentation by recycling yeast cells (Patil *et al.*, 1989).

Patil and Patil (1989) found that top and bottom yeasts together accelerate ethanol production in cane molasses fermentation. Chen and Mou (1990) studied pilot-scale multi-stage multi-feeding mutinous ethanol fermentation using non-sterile cane molasses. The effluent ethanol concentration, overall volumetric productivity and sugar conversion yield averaged 8.54% (v/v), 5.35 g/l-hr and 92.4% of theoretical, respectively.

b) Whey

It is the liquid separated from the curds during cheese making. Earlier, more than half of the whey was dumped away as waste. But due to many innovative uses of whey through microbial fermentation in recent times, it is no longer considered to be a waste product of dairy industry. With an increase in production of cheese and coagulated milk products in India, the processing of whey into any product of industrial importance particularly alcohol, organic acid and beverages will be economically profitable (Gandhi, 1989).

Whey seemed a likely source of alcohol, since it is probably as cheap as any source of fermentable sugar, if a sufficient supply is readily and locally available. Thus, whey as raw material to produce ethyl alcohol was also worked on by Rogosa *et al.*, (1947).

Mann (1980) reviewed the production of alcohols from whey. Sakrzewski and Zmarlicki (1988) reviewed the ethanolic fermentation in whey and whey molasses mixtures. Bacova *et al.*, (1986) have described the technology of alcohol production from whey.

c) Sugar beet

Nain and Rana (1988) conducted nutrient optimization studies for ethanol production from sugar beet juice by *Saccharomyces cerevisiae*. Cochet *et al.*, (1988) demonstrated the feasibility of solid-state fermentation on sugar-beet.

Industrial beet molasses worts for alcoholic fermentation are also good substrates for the growth of some bacteria, especially lactic acid bacteria. The effects of lactic acid on yeast fermentation parameters during alcoholic fermentation of beet molasses was studied by Ngang *et al.*, (1989). Morgan *et al.*,

(1989) worked on solid-state fermentation of sugar-beet for the purpose of fuel-alcohol production.

d) Banana

Acid saccharification and alcohol fermentation of unripe banana fruit has been reported by Pontiveros *et al.*, (1978). Saccharification of the banana peels was carried out by acid, enzyme and steam to optimize the conditions of hydrolysis of the waste banana to reducing sugars. The saccharified material was fermented for alcohol production by *Saccharomyces cerevisiae* (Tewari *et al.*, 1986).

e) Apple

Hang *et al.*, (1981) described production of ethanol from apple pomace with a Montrachet strain of *Saccharomyces cerevisiae*. More than 43g of alcohol could be produced per Kg. of apple pomace fermented at 30 °C in 24 hr.

Miller *et al.*, (1982) worked on saccharification and ethanol fermentation of apple pomace, which is an abundant waste product and presents expensive disposal problem. Dallmann *et al.*, (1987) have reported continuous fermentation of apple juice by immobilized yeast cells.

f) Grape

Hang *et al.*, (1986) used grape pomace as a substrate for the production of ethanol under solid-stat, fermentation conditions. The yield of ethanol amounted to greater than 80 percent of the theoretical, based on the fermentable sugar consumed.

g) Pineapple

A process for the bio-utilization of pineapple waste for ethanol generation has been developed by Tewari *et al.*, (1987).

h) Cassava

Menezes and Lomo (1976) produced alcohol from saccharified cassava by fermentation and used it in fuels. Kunhi et al., (1980) studied the production of alcohol from saccharified waste residue of cassava and revealed that material enriched with mineral salts and nitrogen increases the alcohol production.

Ho and Ghazali (1986) worked on simultaneous saccharification and fermentation of cassava starch to glucose and alcohol by immobilized *Zymomonas mobilis* and immobilized glucoamylase. Akpan et al., (1988) have reported the production of ethanol from cassava whey.

i) Cactus

Retamal et al., (1987) reported ethanol production by fermentation of fruits and cladodes of prickly pear cactus [*Opuntia ficus-indica* (L.) Miller].

j) Water Hyacinth

Kahlon and Kumar (1987) have given the simulation of fermentation conditions for ethanol production from water-hyacinth.

III. Factors influencing fermentation

The factors effecting the process of alcohol fermentation and their optimal control have been reviewed by Abou-Zeid and Farid (1980). The quantitative effects of carbohydrate levels, degree of initial saccharification, glucoamylase dosage, temperature and fermentation temperature were investigated using a Box-Wilson central composite design with *Saccharomyces cerevisiae* ATCC 4126, it was reported that the use of a partially saccharified starch substrate markedly increased yields and attainable alcohol levels. The optimum temperature has been 36 °C (Bowman and Geiger, 1984).

a) Effect of Carbon Sources

Cason *et al.,* (1987) have reported the pitching rates related to Glucose and fructose utilization in *Saccharomyces cerevisiae*. Cason *et al.,* (1987) have also reviewed the differing rates of fructose and glucose utilization in *Saccharomyces cerevisiae*. Fructose is utilized slower than glucose when the two sugars are fermented separately.

Gadd (1988) studied carbon nutrition and metabolism in fungi. Different carbohydrates, mostly polysaccharides, were studied for their effect on ethanol production from cane molasses under batch fermentation conditions using industrial yeast strains, *Saccharomyces cerevisiae* NCIM 3526 and *S. uvarum* NCIM 3509. There is a marked increase in the rate of ethanol production in the presence of polysaccharides like chitin, xylan, and acacia gum at 0.2 percent concentration (Patil and Patil 1989).

b) Effect of Nitrogen Sources

Mullins and Nesmith (1987) showed acceleration of rate of ethanol fermentation by addition of nitrogen in high tannin grain sorghum. The effect of media sterilization and of varying source and concentration of sugar and nitrogen on alcohol production by *Saccharomyces cerevisiae* strains was studied by Halos *et al.,* (1987).

c) Effect of Temperature

Fermentation temperature is one of the most important factors in ethanol formation as it exerts a profound effect on all aspects of growth and survival.

Van Uden (1984) reported that ethanol and other alkanols suppress the maximum and the optimum temperature of growth of *S. cerevisiae*. He discussed the effects of ethanol on the temperature variations of viability growth in yeast.

Borrego et al., (1987) studied effect of temperature and long-term operation on passively immobilized *Zymomonas mobilis* for continuous ethanol production. Richter and Becker (1987) described the effect of temperature on microbial ethanol production. The temperature profile curve of ethanol production of the yeast *S. cerevisiae* was presented.

The analysis of kinetics of ethanol fermentation with *Z. mobilis* considering temperature effect was done by Shih-Yow Huang and Jyn Chern Chen (1988).

Yamamura et al., (1988) studied the effects of elevated temperature on growth, respiratory deficient mutation, respiratory activity and ethanol production in yeast. The effect of temperature on growth and ethanol tolerance of yeasts during wine fermentation was studied by Fleet et al., (1989).

d) Effect of pH

Roberts (1980) reported a pH of 3.5 to be optimum for maximum glucose utilization efficiency. Parsons et al., (1987) have reported an unexpected pH related inhibition of yeast fermentation in a low dilution rate. A higher volumetric rate of ethanol production occurred at lower pH values (2.8 to 3.2) suggesting a low optimum pH.

Borrego and Obon (1988) studied the pH influence on ethanol production and retained biomass in a passively immobilized *Zymomonas mobilis* system. The effect of pH on growth and ethanol production by *Zymomonas* has been described by Lawford et al., (1988). The combined effect of acetic acid, pH and ethanol on intracellular pH of fermenting yeast was studied by Pampulha and Loureiro-Dias (1989). It was noted that for all external pH values tested, the internal pH was 7.0-7.2 in the absence of inhibitors.

Lawford and Ruggiero (1990) worked on studying the effect of pH on maintenance and growth-associated metabolism during production of fuel alcohol by *Zymomonas*.

e) Effect of SO_2

Suitable doses of sulphur dioxide (SO_2), an antioxidant, were found to check the oxidative browning. Use of potassium meta bisulfite to control bacterial contaminants during fermentation of fodder beet cubes for fuel ethanol was reported by Gibbons and Westby (1986). Ough and Crowell (1987) reported that pretreatment of juice with SO_2 helped preserve good color and sensory attributes of the wines. Nakamura et al., (1989) determined free sulphite in wine, making use of a microbial sensor. Angelino et al., (1989) studied activity of sulphate-metabolizing enzymes and SO_2 formation during main fermentation.

f) Effect of substrate concentration

Devine and Slaughter (1980) studied the effect of medium composition on the production of ethanol by *S. cerevisiae*. Richter and Becker (1985) studied the influence of sucrose concentration on the specific ethanol production rate during batch processes using *S. cerevisiae Hansen*. It was found that both the decreases of fermentation activity of the cells caused by sucrose and ethanol have an additional relation to each other.

Kaeppeli and Sonnleitner (1986) reported the regulation of sugar metabolism in *Saccharomyces* type of yeast. Continuous culture experiments revealed that oxidative glucose metabolism is possible at two growth rates. The type of glucose metabolism was found to depend upon the respiratory capacity of the cells.

g) Effect of alcohol accumulation: ethanol tolerance

Bechard *et al.*, (1987) investigated the toxicity effects of alcohols on *S. cerevisiae*. They examined the inhibitory behavior of ethanol through systematic variation of glucose and alcohol concentration. The results show non-competitive inhibition of glucose metabolism for low ethanol concentration. Jimenez and Benitex (1987) reported adaption of yeast cell membranes to ethanol.

D'Amore *et al.*, (1987) studied the effect of osmotic pressure on the intracellular accumulation of ethanol in *S. cerevisiae* during fermentation in wort. Ghareib *et al.*, (1988) described ethanol tolerance of *S. cerevisiae* and its relationship to lipid content and composition. Physiological factors such as mode of substrate feeding, intracellular ethanol accumulations, temperature and osmotic pressure, all contribute to the ethanol tolerance of yeast (D'Amore and Stewart 1987).

Toda *et al.*, (1987) studied inhibitory effect of ethanol on ethanol fermentation. Anaerobic growth of *Saccharomyces carlsbergensis* LAM1068 was inhibited completely at the ethanol concentration of P_{mg} = 95 g/l. Fleet and Chong Xiao Gao (1988) reviewed the effects of temperature and pH on the ethanol tolerance of the wine yeasts, *S. cerevisiae*, *Candida stellata* and *Kloeckera apiculata*. Jones (1988) made a study on intracellular ethanol-accumulation and exit from yeast and other cells.

Leite and Franca (1988) conducted a preliminary study on the effect of the addition of ethanol to the alcoholic fermentation carried out by *S. cerevisiae* F1. D'Amore and Panchal (1988) reported osmotic pressure effects and intracellular accumulation of ethanol in yeast during fermentation. Ramos and Madeira-Lopes (1990) studied the effects of acetic acid on the temperature profile of ethanol tolerance in *S. cerevisiae*.

h) Growth inhibition

Jones and Greenfield (1987) studied specific and non-specific inhibitory effects of ethanol on yeast growth. The inhibition of growth of yeast by octanoic or decanoic acids was evaluated in *S. cerevisiae* and *Kluyveromyces marxianus* in association with ethanol. (Viegas *et al.*, 1989). Pampulha and Loureiro (1989) studied the interaction of the effects of acetic acid and ethanol on inhibition of fermentation in *S. cerevisiae*.

i) Continuous Ethanol Production

Todder (1985) described a patent for a continuous method of preparing alcohol. The method consists of continuously fermenting using micro-organisms. Shankar *et al.*, (1985) studied continuous ethanol production by *S. uvarum* immobilized in a low-gelling temperature agarose in a packed bed reactor at 30 °C using sugarcane molasses as feed.

Sam and St. Bringer-Meyer (1987) reported continuous ethanol production by *Z. mobilis* on an industrial scale. Hill and Robinson (1988) studied morphological behavior of *S. cerevisiae* during continuous fermentation. A model solid substrate was developed, consisting of cassava starch and other nutrients by Mitchell *et al.*, (1988). Salzbrunn *et al.*, (1989) described a method of continuously producing ethanol from sugar-containing substrates comprising fermentation of the sugar in said substrate by a flocculating strain of *Z. mobilis* cells under anaerobic conditions.

Bajpai *et al.,* (1989) reviewed continuous ethanol production using immobilized cells of high-ethanol-producing yeast. Pasari *et al.,* (1989) gave a model for continuous fermentations with amylolytic yeasts.

j) Microorganisms for ethanol production

For the industrial production of ethanol, yeasts are the only microorganisms being used currently. Yeasts produce ethanol with very high selectivity and are very hardy and large as compared to bacteria. The bacterium *Z. mobilis* ferments glucose to ethanol with a typical rate 5-20 percent higher than for most yeasts, but is less ethanol tolerant. The small bacterium is also difficult to centrifuge (Maiorella, 1984).

The fermentation of sucrose based raw materials has been studied using immobilized cells of *Z. mobilis* in a lab-scale bioreactor (Grote and Rogers, 1985). De Franca *et al.,* (1986) reported alcoholic fermentation of mandioc flour by *Zymomonas sp.* Deshpande *et al.,* (1986) reported direct conversion of cellulose to ethanol by *Neurospora crassa*. Rao and Mutharasan (1986) studied alcohol production by *Clostridium acetobutylicum* induced by methyl viologen.

Ghommidh and Bu'lock (1988) worked on ethanol production with artificially flocculated *Zymomonas* cells. The use of wheat bran as a nutritive supplement for the production of ethanol by *Z. mobilis* was described by Shamala and Sreekantiah (1988). Lawford (1988) described ethanol production by high performance bacterial fermentation. The effect of high glucose concentrations on continuous ethanol production by passively immobilized *Z. mobilis* cells was studied by Castellar *et al.*, (1989).

Lawford (1989) described a continuous process for ethanol rial fermentation. Millichip (1989) studied ethanol production by *Zymomonas* cultures in yeast-conditioned media. The ethanol fermentation by *Z. mobilis* ATCC 10988 in repeated batch was described by Agrawal and Veeramallu (1990).

IV. Production of wines

Wine is a beverage resulting from the fermentation by yeasts Of the juice of certain fruits with appropriate processing and additions. (Amerine and Singleton, 1968).

The use of wine goes back to time immemorial. The Bible, Homer's epic, Egyptian documents etc. mention it. Somras (Wine) is our Vedic drink (Tewari, 1980). However it was time of the middle ages when the alchemists discovered the active principle ethanol. At the end of the 17th century Leeuwenhoek described the yeasts in grape musts and worts, but he established no relationship between yeasts and fermentations. A century later Lavoisier published the first scientific work on fermentation which he considered a purely chemical phenomenon. It was in 1836 that Cagnard-Latour proved the role of yeasts, living organisms which cause biochemical transformations. Since 1950 the development of chemical, chromatographic and enzymatic techniques has led to more sophisticated studies. (Lafourcade, 1983).

As a result wine has deeply penetrated the social fabric and culture of times and countries from which we spring. (Amerine and Houghton 1968). Tewari *et al.*, (1987) reported the utilization of sub-standard pears for the production of wines as food and medicine. A method for making an acceptable quality of plum wine has been reported by Vyas and Joshi (1982) and Tewari *et al.,* (1988). Utilization of pineapple waste for wine making has been reported by Alian and Musenge (1970) and Tewari *et al.,* (1987).

Minarik (1985) has reported some microbiological and biotechnological problems in wine making. Wine from banana has been chemically and seasonally analyzed by Stein (1986). Banana peels have been utilized for the production of ethanol by Tewari *et al.,* (1986).

Wines and vinegars are being used as food and medicine since ages (Tewari and Gupta, 1978). Wine from *M. charantia* has medicinal value for diabetes. Tewari (1979, 1981 and 1986). A manual for diabetics has been published by Tewari (1979). Feasibility of processing of grapes in Punjab state and the establishment of experimental winery, Punjab Marketing Federation, Chandigarh has been reported by Tewari (1978). There has also been a report on the establishment of pilot scale grape processing plant for wines and brandy in Punjab (Tewari, 1978).

Biological qualities of grapes grown in Punjab state have been utilized for the production of wines by Tewari *et al.,* (1978). Substantial pear fruit has been successfully utilized for the production of commercial wines and has been awarded first prize by the Punjab State International Society (Tewari *et al.,* 1987).

Obisanya *et al.,* (1987) have produced wine from mango (Mangifera indica L.) using *Saccharomyces* and *Schizosaccharomyces* species isolated from palm wine. Reed and Nagodawithana (1988) have described the technology of yeast usage in wine making. Laude *et al.,* (1987) described a process for thermally controlling the wine-making process. Lee and Kime (1990) showed that the production of wine from grapes could be improved by addition of honey and SO_2 in a total amount effective to inhibit browning discoloration. Lembke et al., (1989) gave a process for the production of sparkling wine.

V. Dehydration of Ethanol for fuel

The water bulk present in the fermented liquid can be readily separated from the alcohol by fractional distillation due to considerable difference in boiling points (100 °C and 78-32 °C). But it is difficult to obtain complete separation of two liquids owing to the formation of boiling azeotrope containing 95.57% alcohol and 4.43 percent water at 73.15 °C. The boiling point difference between the azeotrope and the pure alcohol is too small to permit separation.

Calcium oxide is perhaps the earliest known solid dehydrating agent for production of absolute alcohol and was practiced for over a hundred years on laboratory scale and later adopted to industrial use.

Venugopal et al., (1964) studied the performance of different solid desiccants (anhydrous) $CaSO_4$, Na_2, SO_4, alumina, $MgSO_4$, silica gel, sodium and potassium acetates and amberlite IR-12. Their analysis revealed that chemical compounds subjected to calcination and having narrow pore distribution cannot be effective desiccant while compounds subjected to precipitation, flocculation and drying to considerate temperatures function as effective desiccants. Anhydrous $CaSO_4$ and alumina were found to be the only suitable desiccants for effective dehydration, and fixed bed gave better performance as compared to fluidized bed. The aqueous alcohol produced from waste potatoes was dehydrated by $MgSO_4 \cdot 7H_2O$ and calcium chloride $CaCl_2 \cdot 6H_2O$ by Tewari et al., (1982, 1983).

VI. Immobilization of Yeasts

Marwaha et al., (1985) reviewed immobilization of yeasts. An immobilization technique of yeast cells by using polyethylene glycol-diacrylate (PEG-DA) and 2-hydroxyethyl acrylate (HEA) has been developed for continuous ethanol production by Maeda et al., (1985). Techniques for immobilizing cells are application oriented and include encapsulation, covalent or ionic attachment to solid supports, entrapment in gelatinous matrices and encapsulation in membranes. Immobilized cell systems are efficient and have the potential of high-volume productivities. In Japan 20 KL pilot fermenters with immobilized growing yeast cells have been operating for 6 months with continuous ethanol production at 12 KL/day. (Bothast and Slininger, 1984).

Continuous ethanol production by yeast cells immobilized in a pure gelatin matrix, was reported by Sivaraman et al., (1982). Yeast cells immobilized in pectin gel have no significant changes in their biological activity. (Navarro et al., 1983). The ethanol production rate was found to be negatively affected by the diameter of the beads when the cell concentration in them was high.

Growing cells of S. cerevisiae immobilized in calcium alginate gel beads have been employed in fluidized bed reactors for continuous ethanol fermentation from cane-molasses and other sugar sources (Nagashima et al., 1984). Studies on the addition of different ratios of sand in alginate immobilized S. formosensis conducted by Fang et al., (1984) have increased the efficiency of alcoholic fermentation. Beads of porous agar with entrapped yeast cells have been used for the continuous fermentation of sugar cane molasses to ethanol (Rao et al., 1981).

The immobilization of whole cells is a technique that can be used in several production processes, among them alcoholic fermentation. This study was done by Nunez and Lema (1987). By using a column packed with immobilized S. cerevisiae cells entrapped in a polyacrylamide gel lattice, conditions for continuous production of ethanol were investigated by Baranaik et al., 1987. A procedure for immobilization of S. uvarum cells in porous beads of polyacrylamide gel for ethanolic fermentation was also described by Pundle et al., in 1988. Phani et al., (1988) reported immobilization of S. cerevisiae in calcium alginate gel and its application to bottle fermented sparkling wine production.

Bajpai et al., (1988) reported rapid production of ethanol in high concentration by immobilized cells of S. cerevisiae through soya flour supplementation. The effect of the organic and inorganic matrices on the performance of ethanol fermentation by S. bayanus was tested by Passarinho et al., (1989). Theoretical and practical viewpoints for production of alcohol by immobilized yeasts and bacteria have been discussed by Ivanova et al., (1989).

Amin and Doelle (1989) designed a vertical rotating immobilized reactor of the bacterium *Zymomonas mobilis* for stable long term continuous ethanol production.

Chithra and Baradarajan (1989) conducted studies on co-immobilization of amyloglucosidase and S. cerevisiae for direct conversion of starch to ethanol. A mathematical model was developed by Jinescu et al., (1989), regarding the immobilized living yeast cell reactor for sugar bioconversion to ethanol. The model composed of a system of ordinary differential equations (ODEs) enables the computation of parameters involved in the steady state reactor behavior.

Hoshino et al., (1989) reviewed repeated batch conversion of raw starch to ethanol using amylase immobilized on a reversible soluble-auto precipitating carrier and flocculating yeast cells. Richter et al., (1990) reported ethanolic fermentation with S. cerevisiae cells immobilized in pectate gel.

Chapter III – MATERIALS AND METHODS

3.1 Substrate

The fruit, Mango (Mangifera indica var. Dussehri) used for This study was collected from the local market, Ludhiana. The substandard fruits were categorized as immature, brown coloration, ruptured, and damaged by birds as shown in Fig. 1-4.

3.2 Micro-organisms

Saccharomyces cerevisiae var. ellipsoideus used in the study was obtained from the culture collection, Department of Microbiology, Punjab Agricultural University, Ludhiana.

The yeast culture was maintained on Glucose yeast extract medium (Tuite, 1969) having the following composition:

Glucose	10.0 g
Yeast extract	5.0 g
Peptone	5.0 g
Agar	20.0 g
Distilled water	1,000 ml
pH	5.0

The yeast culture was subcultured at regular intervals and maintained on GYE slants stored at 4 °C.

Fig 1: Immature Mango Fruit

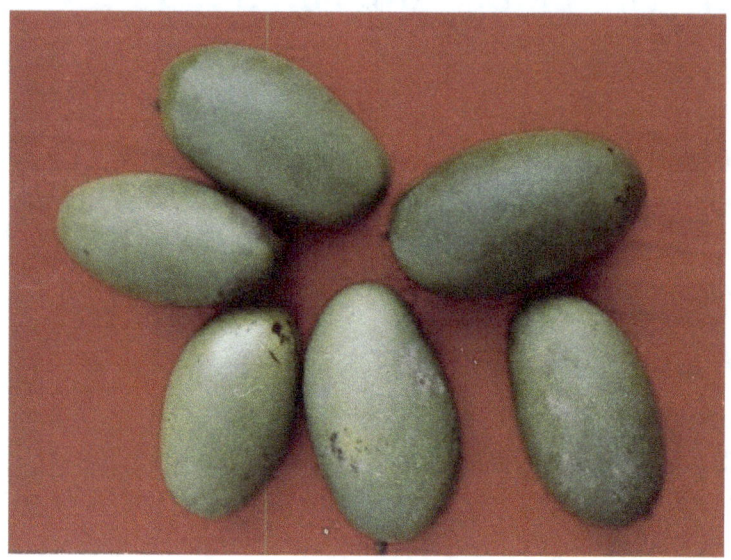

Fig 2: Discolored Mango Fruit

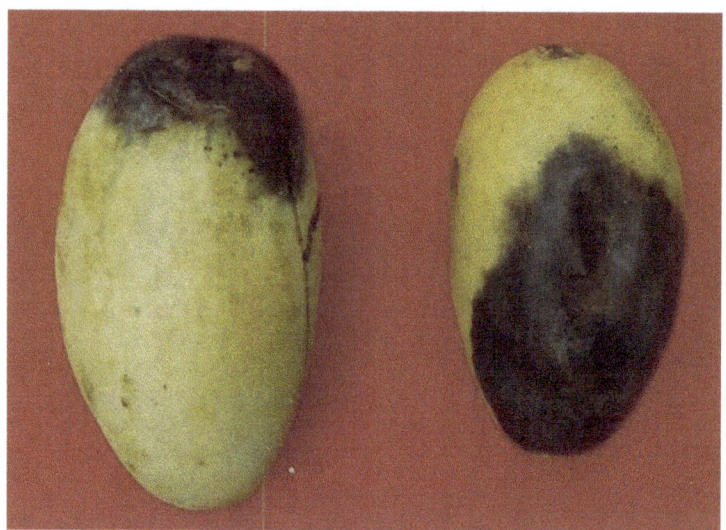

Fig 3: Ruptured Mango Fruit

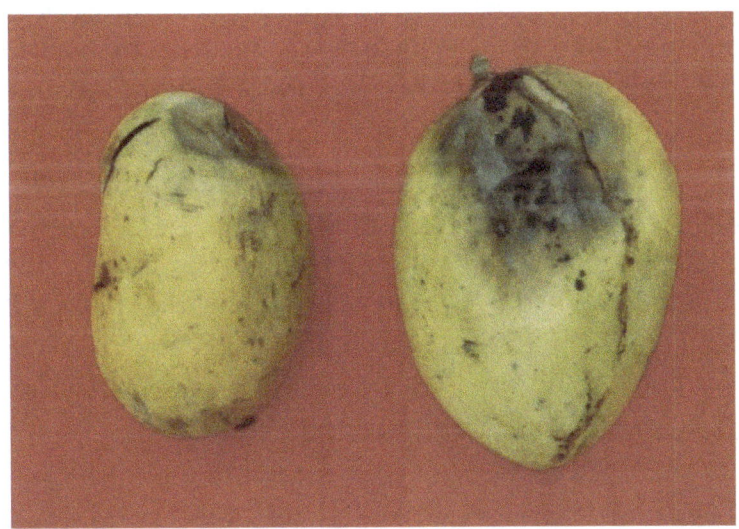

Fig 4: Mango Fruit Damaged by Birds

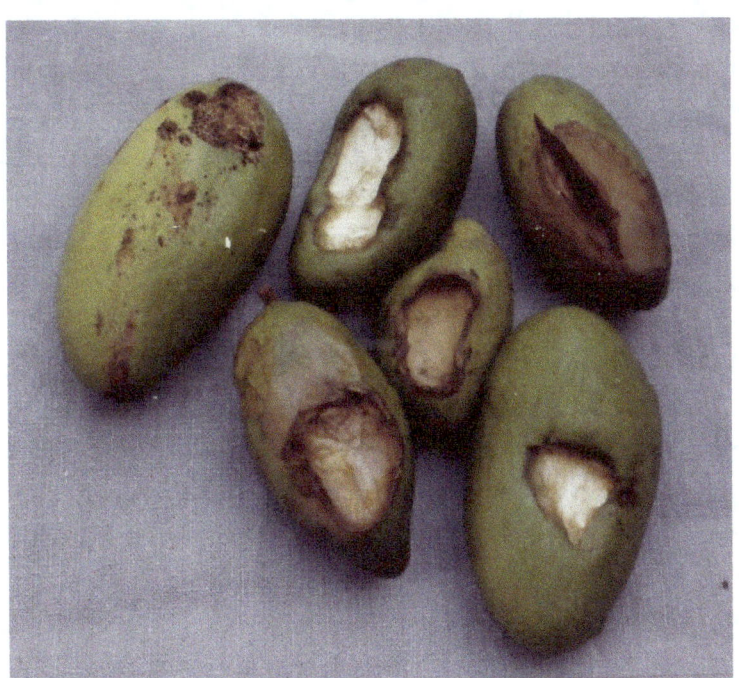

3.3 Extraction and Treatment of Juice

The fruits were properly washed under tap water and kept at room temperature. The juice was extracted manually. The pulp of each fruit was softened by pressing between the palms of the hands and then it was squeezed out. Potassium metabisulfite (KMS) @ 50 ppm was added to it to prevent contamination. The utensils were thoroughly washed with boiling hot water prior to use. Diluted the mango juice by adding four times its weight of water. The juice was analyzed for TSS, reducing sugars, total acids, volatile acids and pH. The fruit juice was adjusted to required °Brix using cane sugar syrup and it was pasteurized at 60 °C for 20 minutes.

3.4 Ethanol Fermentation
a) Preparation of inoculum:

The inoculum was prepared by inoculating 100 ml of glucose yeast extract broth, with loopful of 20hr old actively growing culture of yeast. (*S. cerevisiae*). The 250ml Erlenmeyer flasks were incubated to a rotary shaker (120 rpm) at 28 °C for 20 hrs. The inoculum thus prepared was used to inoculate the fruit juice which was then incubated for 24 hours. The contents were used as starter culture to carry out the ethanol fermentation.

b) Fermentation of the Juice:

The fermentation was carried out in 250ml Erlenmeyer flasks. 100ml of pasteurized juice, which was standardized to 20 °Brix was taken in each of these flasks. The initial Brix was noted using a refractometer. The fruit **must** was then inoculated with starter culture of *S. cerevisiae* var. ellipsoideus (@ 15% v/v) and the fermentation was carried out at 30 ± 2 °C. The contents were shaken 3-4 times a day. The fall in brix was noted at specific intervals, regularly with the help of Erma Hand Refractometer. The observations were made till steady state values were obtained. The product was analyzed for ethyl alcohol (% v/v).

Since the inoculum level, pH, sugar concentration, temperature and SO_2, have an impact on fermentation, so their effects were evaluated for sufficient fermentation. All the experiments in the present investigation were performed in duplicates.

i. Inoculum level

To study the effect of inoculum concentration on ethanol production, the culture of *S. cerevisiae* var. ellipsoideus was inoculated @ 8.0, 10.0, 12.0 and 15.0 percent in 250ml flasks containing 100ml standard fruit mash. It was then incubated at 30 ± 2 °C.

ii. Effect of Total Soluble Solids

The initial brix of the fruit juice was adjusted to 8, 10, 12, 15, 18 and 20°B, with the help of cane sugar to study the effect of total soluble solids on the alcoholic fermentation.

iii. Effect of pH

The fruit **must** was adjusted to pH 4.0, 4.5, 5.0, and 5.5 to study the effect of pH on alcoholic fermentation. The pH was adjusted by use of liquid ammonia and phosphoric acid (2% each).

iv. Effect of SO_2

The effect of sulphur dioxide on alcohol fermentation was studied by adding Potassium metabisulfite (KMS) at the conc. of 50, 80, 100 and 125 ppm.

v. Effect of temperature

Keeping rest of the conditions optimum the fermentation was carried out at 25 ± 2 °C, 30 ± 2 °C and room temperature (29-42 °C).

Clarification of Wine

The fermented mash was stored at 4 °C for 2-3 days, was siphoned off to remove settled dead yeast cells and other must sediments. The wine was further clarified by resiphoning.

3.5 Analysis
i. Total Soluble Solids (TSS)

The TSS (°Brix) of juice and wine were determined by using Erma hand Refractometer.

ii. pH

The pH was determined by pH meter (Elico). The pH meter was standardized to pH 4.0 with a standard buffer solution before use.

iii. Total acidity (Amerine *et al.,* 1980)
Reagents

    a. Sodium hydroxide (0.1N): 4.0g of sodium hydroxide pellets were dissolved in 1,000 ml of distilled water.

    b. Phenolphthalein indicator (1%): Dissolve 1 g of phenolphthalein in 100ml of ethanol.

Procedure:

Pipetted 5ml of sample, diluted it to 50ml using distilled water. Then added 2-3 drops of phenolphthalein indicator. Titrated it with 0.1 N NaOH, adding it dropwise from burette till one drop gives the end point i.e. from colorless to pink. Recorded the amount of alkali used.

Calculations:
1 ml of 0.1 N NaOH = 0.015 g tartaric acid

$$\text{Total acidity (\% w/v)} = \frac{\text{Vol. of 0.1 N NaOH used} \times 0.015 \times 100}{5}$$

iv. Volatile Acidity (Amerine *et al.*, 1980)
Reagents
  a. Sodium hydroxide (0.1N)

  b. Phenolphthalein indicator (1%)

Procedure

To estimate volatile acidity the apparatus required is a 2,000ml wide mouthed boiling flask, an inner cylindrical glass tube fitted inside the boiling flask by a wide rubber stopper and liebig condenser connected vertically to the glass tubing. The estimation was done by done by taking about 1 liter of distilled water which was heated to boiling for 2-3 minutes. Five milliliters of juice or wine sample was introduced into the inner tube using a pipette. The rubber stopper connecting the inner tube to the condenser was replaced. The contents were boiled and over 100ml of distillate was collected in 250ml previously marked conical flask. Now, to the distillate 2-3 drops of phenolphthalein indicator was added. The resultant solution was titrated to a light pink color using 0.1 N NaOH.

Calculations:
1 ml of 0.1 N NaOH = 0.006 g acetic acid

$$\text{\% Volatile acidity (w/v)} = \frac{\text{Vol. of 0.1 N NaOH used} \times 0.006 \times 100}{\text{volume of sample}}$$

v. Estimation of reducing sugars (Miller, 1959)

Reagents

a. Dinitrosalicylic acid (DNS) reagent: 10g of 3,5 dinitrosalicylic acid, 2.0g phenol and 0.5g sodium sulfite were dissolved in 500ml of one percent sodium hydroxide solution. The volume was then made to one liter with alkaline solution.

b. Sodium-potassium tartrate (Rochelle Salt) solution: 40g of Sodium-potassium tartrate were dissolved in distilled water and the volume made to 100 ml.

Procedure

The experiment was conducted in duplicates. Test-tubes containing 3ml of samples and 3ml of DNS reagent were heated for 15min. in boiling water bath. Then 1ml of Rochelle salt solution was added to each tube and cooled to room-temperature. Using Bausch and Lomb Spectronic-20, the optical density was measured at 575 nm. A control was prepared for each experiment. Standard curve was prepared by taking 0.1 to 1.0 mg/ml of glucose.

vi. Ethanol Estimation

Reagents:

a. Potassium Dichromate solution: To 200ml distilled water add 16.8gm Potassium dichromate and dissolve it. Now place it in a water bath and add 162.5ml H_2SO_4 slowly. Keep cooling side by side. Make the volume to 500 ml.

Procedure:

A standard curve was prepared by using standard solution of ethanol containing 0, 2, 4, 6, 8, 10 and 12% (v/v) ethanol in distilled water.

For determining the ethanol content of fermented wash, 1ml of it was taken in 500ml Pyrex distillation flask and 30ml of distilled water was added. 20ml of the distillate was collected in 50ml volumetric flask containing 25ml of $K_2Cr_2O_7$ solution. The flasks were then kept in a water bath maintained at 60 °C for 20min. They were then cooled to room temperature and the volume made to 50ml. 5ml of this was taken and diluted with 5ml of distilled water and optical density was recorded at 600nm on Spectronic-20.

Calculations:

$$\text{Fermentation efficiency} = \frac{\text{Actual recovery}}{\text{theoretical recovery}} \times 100$$

Theoretical Recovery = Total Fermentable Sugars x 0.51

Actual Recovery = Actual ethanol produced

vii. Wine analysis and evaluation

The wine samples were analyzed for total soluble solids, pH, reducing sugars, volatile acidity and ethanol. The mango wine was evaluated by using the wine score card.

viii. Dehydration of Aqueous ethanol

The dehydration of 95 percent alcohol was done by $CaCl_2.6H_2O$. (18 g/100 ml, w/v). Calcium chloride was added to 95 percent alcohol in 500ml conical flask. The mouths of flasks were closed and then they were kept on shaker for two hours. Thereafter the mixtures were transferred to the distillation flask and the alcohol was estimated in the distillate by alcoholometer.

Chapter IV – RESULTS AND DISCUSSION

The results of various experiments conducted to optimize the fermentation conditions for ethanol production are discussed under the following headings:

1. Composition of mango juice

2. Ethanol fermentation

3. Analysis and evaluation of mango wine

4. Dehydration of aqueous ethanol for the production of fuel alcohol.

1. Composition of Mango Juice

Table 1: Composition of mango juice* (***Var. Dussehri***)

Total Soluble Solids (TSS, °Brix)	6.8
Reducing Sugars (g%)	5.4
Total Acids (% Tartaric acid)	0.50
Volatile acids (% Acetic acid)	0.001
Potassium metabisulphite (ppm)	50.0
pH	5.2
*Mango juice diluted with water (@1:4 w/v)	

2. Ethanol Fermentation

Saccharomyces cerevisiae var ellipsoideus was used for alcoholic fermentation of mango juice. The results of the effect of various fermentation parameters such as total soluble solids, fermentation temperature, pH and concentration of inoculum on ethanol production have been discussed (Tables: 2 to 8)

2.1 Total Soluble Solids (TSS) Vs Alcoholic Fermentation:

The total soluble solids in the fruit juice were varied from 8° to 20 °Brix to study its effect on ethanol production. The results of the effect of total soluble solids on ethanol fermentation are presented in Table 2.

The fermentation completed within 36 to 84 hours in all the treatments. The fermentation completed within 36 hrs in the control treatment whereas it completed within 48, 48, 60, 84, 84 and 72 hrs with initial TSS of 8, 10, 12, 15, 18 and 20 °B respectively. Final TSS has been found to be 2.4 °B in all the treatments. About 50 percent of the substrate was utilized by the yeast for its conversion to ethanol within 24 hrs of fermentation with initial TSS of 8° to 15 °B and in the control treatment as well. The fermentation period increased with further increase in initial substrate concentration. Substrate (60 percent) was utilized within 36 hrs of fermentation at 18° and 20 °B.

More than 75 percent of the substrate was converted to ethanol within 48 hrs with initial TSS (10° and 20 °B) and within 60 hrs with initial TSS of 12 and 15 °B. The total substrate utilized in the case of the control experiment was only about 65 percent. The substrate utilization gradually increased with increase in the initial TSS.

The total substrate utilization was 70, 76, 80, 84, 86.7 and 88 percent with the initial TSS of 8, 10, 12, 15, 18 and 20 °Brix respectively in the experiment to study the effect of total soluble solids on ethanol fermentation.

Neelam (1987) has reported 20 °B to be optimum for efficient alcoholic fermentation of pear juice. Anshula (1987) has reported 15 °B to be optimum for fermentation of jamun. Cheema (1989) has reported TSS (10 °B) as optimum for fermentation of guava. Tewari et al., (1987) have reported 22 °B to be optimum for apple juice fermentation. Ribereau - Gayon (1984) gave reasons that cessation of fermentation by *S. cerevisiae* in a medium rich in sugar was not due to an inhibition of the activities of hexokinase and dehydrogenase.

Lafon - Lafourcade (1983) has clarified the reasons for decreased ability of yeast for complete utilization of sugars with increase in sugar concentration at initial stages. He stated that in **musts** with elevated levels of sugars the final part of fermentation is conducted by cells in the decline phase, where their metabolic activity decreases and this leads to premature cessation of fermentation. Panchal and Stewart (1980) also reported that when the substrate concentration increases beyond 25 percent, the effect of osmotic pressure becomes pronounced which seriously affects fermentation efficiency and leads to decreased ethanol production.

Richter and Becker (1985) studied the influence of sucrose concentration on the specific ethanol production rate during batch processes using *S. cerevisiae*. They have reported that decrease in fermentation activity of the cells caused by sucrose and ethanol have an additional relation to each other. It was also taken into consideration that the maximum ethanol concentration cannot be realized at high substrate concentration in a batch process as compared to it, sucrose concentration below 100 g/l did not inhibit ethanol production.

Table 2: TSS vs Alcoholic Fermentation

Fermentation period (hr)	TSS °B						
	6.8	8.0	10.0	12.0	15.0	18.0	20.0
0	6.8	8.0	10.0	12.0	15.0	18.0	20.0
12	5.2	6.2	8.6	9.4	12.8	15.8	17.8
24	3.2	4.0	5.0	5.6	7.0	11.0	13.2
36	2.4	2.6	4.0	3.4	5.2	7.2	8.0
48	2.4	2.4	2.4	3.4	4.2	3.6	4.0
60	2.4	2.4	2.4	2.4	3.2	3.2	2.8
72	2.4	2.4	2.4	2.4	2.8	2.8	2.4
84	2.4	2.4	2.4	2.4	2.4	2.4	2.4

Fermentation Conditions:
    Temperature: 30 ± 2 °C
    Inoculum @: 15% (v/v)
    pH   : 5.2

It may be concluded from the results of the experiment on the effect of total soluble solids on ethanol production that initial TSS (20 °B) is optimum for alcoholic fermentation of mango juice. Initial TSS (20 °B) was maintained for further studies.

2.2 Inoculum Concentration vs Alcoholic Fermentation:

The results in Table 3 depict the effect of inoculum level (8-15% v/v) of *S. cerevisiae* var ellipsoideus on alcoholic fermentation of mango juice.

It has been observed that with 15 percent (v/v) inoculum level the fermentation was efficient, as the TSS at 84 hrs of fermentation was 2.4 °Brix, whereas at the same time for 8, 10, and 12 percent (v/v) Inoculum it was 4.2, 3.2 and 3.2 °B respectively. About 50 percent of the substrate was utilized at 36 hrs of fermentation with 12 and 15 percent (v/v) inoculum concentration, while the same amount of substrate was utilized within 60 and 48 hrs at 8 and 10 percent (v/v) inoculum level respectively. The final TSS in all the treatments has been found to be 2.4 °B. More than 75 percent of the substrate was utilized by yeast within 84, 72, 60 and 48 hrs with inoculum levels 8, 10, 12,and 15 percent (v/v) respectively. The fermentation was continued till 120 hrs i.e. till constant values of TSS were attained.

Tewari *et al.*, (1987) have reported an inoculum of *S. cerevisiae* @ 10.0 percent (v/v) to be optimum for alcoholic fermentation of juices from jamun, two varieties of plums and apples. Neelam (1987) has reported 10 percent (v/v) inoculum of *S. cerevisiae* for alcoholic fermentation of pear juice. Cheema (1989) reported an inoculum concentration of 10 percent (v/v) as optimum for fermentation of guava. Strehaiano *et al.*, (1983) have reported decrease in fermentation duration with increase in inoculum level. An inoculum concentration of 10 percent (v/v) has been found optimum by these workers for industrial fermentation as it reduces the lag in the initiation of fermentation, fermentation period and reduces the chances of contamination of fermentation media. Moreover, it was observed by Strehaiano *et al.,* (1983) that the application of higher inoculum level (60% v/v), no doubt shortens the fermentation period, but its use makes the process economically non-viable.

Table 3: Inoculum vs Alcoholic Fermentation

Fermentation period (hr)	Inoculum % (v/v)			
	8.0	10.0	12.0	15.0
	TSS °B			
0	20.0	20.0	20.0	20.0
12	18.2	18.2	18.0	18.0
24	16.0	15.0	14.2	13.6
36	12.6	11.4	9.4	8.8
48	11.4	10.0	7.2	4.2
60	8.0	5.2	4.6	3.0
72	6.8	4.4	4.0	2.6
84	4.2	3.2	3.2	2.4
96	3.4	2.8	2.6	2.4
108	2.4	2.4	3.0	2.4
120	2.4	2.4	2.4	2.4

Fermentation Conditions:
    Temperature: 30 ± 2 °C
    Initial TSS   : 20.0 °B
    pH   : 5.2

Similar results have been reported by Ghose and Tyagi (1979), who showed that the fermentation time to produce 12 percent (v/v) ethanol from hydrolysate was lowered as the inoculum concentration was increased. This was explained by the lower extent of cell multiplication at high inoculum levels. Bannerjee et al., (1984) conducted detailed studies to see the effect of inoculum size on ethanol yield using the extract of sugar beet or sweet sorghum for fermentation to ethanol and the results indicated that 10 percent inoculum was most suitable.

Abou Zeid and Reddy (1986) used 12-14 percent yeast inocula and found their results to be comparable and it's only the length of fermentation that is markedly affected. Nain and Rana (1988) established optimum operating conditions for ethanol production from sugar beet juice by *S. cerevisiae*. Optimum inoculum level was found to be 10 percent (v/v).

In the present study the fermentation has been fast at 15 percent (v/v) inoculum. So it may be concluded that 15 percent (v/v) inoculum size is optimum for fermentation of mango juice and this concentration has been used in further experiments to optimize the generation of ethanol from mango.

2.3 Temperature vs Alcoholic Fermentation:

An experiment to ascertain the optimum fermentation temperature for alcoholic fermentation of mango juice has shown that fermentation temperature affected the conversion of sugars to ethanol by *S. cerevisiae*. The fermentation temperatures studied were 25 °C, 30 °C and room temperature (29 – 42 °C). The results of the experiment are presented in Table 4.

The fermentation was continued for 96 hrs till constant TSS was recorded in all the treatments. Fermentation was slow at 25 °C, as compared to fermentation at 30 °C and at room temperature. About 50 percent of the substrate was utilized after 36 hrs of fermentation in all the treatments. At 30 °C fermentation completed within 84 hrs whereas it continued till 96 hrs at 25 °C and at room temperature. Seventy-five percent of the substrate was found to have been utilized by yeast for conversion to ethanol within 48 hrs at 30 °C while the same amount has been utilized within 60 hrs at 25 °C and at room temperature. The final TSS has been 2.4 °Brix in all the treatments.

From these observations it can be summarized that fermentation was optimum at 30 °C.

Table 4: Fermentation Temperature vs Alcoholic Fermentation

Fermentation period (hr)	Fermentation temperature °C		
	25 ± 2	25 ± 2	Room Temp*
	TSS °B		
0	20.0	20.0	20.0
12	17.6	18.0	18.0
24	14.0	13.8	14.2
36	10.2	8.2	9.2
48	6.0	4.0	7.8
60	4.2	3.0	5.0
72	3.0	2.6	3.2
84	2.6	2.4	2.6
96	2.4	2.4	2.4

Fermentation Conditions:
    Initial TSS : 20.0 °B
    Inoculum @: 15% (v/v)
    pH : 5.2
*Room Temperature: 29 – 42 °C

These results are in line within the findings of several workers. Tewari *et al.,* (1985, 1986, 1987 and 1988) have reported a temperature of 30 °C as optimum for alcoholic fermentation of saccharified banana peels and of juice from jamun, plums, apples and grapes. The explanation for premature cessation of fermentation at higher temperature by Nagodawithana and Steinkraus (1976) and Navarro and Durand (1980) is that at higher fermentation temperatures, the inhibitory effect of ethanol is also higher as the ethanol accumulates within the cells due to the resistance to diffusion through cell wall.

Rogosa et al., (1947) have observed maximum fermentation at 37 °C but recommended a fermentation of 33 – 34 °C. Lokendra Singh (1984) reported a temperature of 30 °C to be optimum for fermentation of cellulosic wastes. Neelam (1987) has reported 30 °C as optimum temperature for alcoholic fermentation of pear juice. Cheema (1989) has reported a temperature of 30 °C to be optimum for fermentation of guava. Lee et al., (1980) have reported a temperature of 34 °C optimum for growth while 37-43 °C for maximum specific ethanol production rate. The inhibitory effect of ethanol on growth and specific ethanol production rate was unaffected by the temperature up to 37 °C. However at this temperature ethanol inhibition increased significantly.

Hang et al., (1981) carried out fermentation of apple pomace and observed that sugar consumption and ethanol production was higher at 30 °C. Dombek and Ingram (1986) too observed 30 °C as an optimum temperature for fermentation by S. cerevisiae. Orlowski and Barford (1987) maintained an optimum of 30 °C to conduct their studies on fermentation using S. cerevisice. Richter and Becker (1987) described the effects of temperature on microbial ethanol production.

The maximum specific ethanol formation rate V_o is reached within the temperature limits of 32 °C < T < 36 °C.

The fermentation temperature was maintained at 30 °C for further experiments to be conducted for optimization of other parameters for ethanol fermentation.

2.4 pH vs Alcoholic Fermentation:

The results presented in Table 5 revealed an increase in fermentation rate with an increase in pH from 4.0-5.0 but at pH 5.5 a decrease in fermentation rate was recorded. The fermentation started within 12 hrs in all the treatments. At pH 5.0 the fermentation was completed within 72 hrs whereas at pH 4.0, 4.5 and 5.5 the fermentation was completed at 84, 84 and 96 hrs respectively. The final TSS in all treatments has been observed to be 2.4 °B. Fifty percent of the substrate was utilized at 36 hrs in all the treatments. Fermentation was continued till 96 hrs i.e. till constant values of TSS were obtained.

These observations are in concurrence with the works of Dombek and Ingram (1986) who used medium adjusted to pH 5.0 for fermentation by *S. cerevisiae*. Orlowski and Barford (1987) too maintained a pH of 5.0 to conduct their studies. Grewal (1986), Neelam (1987), Anshula (1987) and Cheema (1989) have recorded a pH range of 4.5-5.0 as optimum for maximum ethanol production from different fruit juices. Prescott and Dunn (1949), Underkofler *et al.,* (1954), Tewari *et al.,* (1983 b, 1985 and 1986) have reported a pH range of 4.0-5.0 optimum for alcoholic fermentation of molasses, grains, saccharified potato mash, saccharified saw dust and plums.

Table 5: pH vs Alcoholic Fermentation

Fermentation period (hr)	pH			
	4.0	4.5	5.0	5.5
	TSS °B			
0	20.0	20.0	20.0	20.0
12	18.2	18.0	17.6	18.2
24	14.0	15.0	14.6	15.6
36	8.2	8.2	8.0	9.0
48	4.0	3.8	3.0	5.0
60	3.2	3.0	2.6	4.0
72	2.6	2.6	2.4	3.0
84	2.4	2.4	2.4	2.8
96	2.4	2.4	2.4	2.4

Fermentation Conditions:
    Initial TSS   : 20.0 °B
    Inoculum @ : 15% (v/v)
    Temperature: 30 ± 2 °C

Rolz et al., (1980) have reported pH 4.5 to be optimum for alcohol production at laboratory scale from sugarcane pieces by the EX-FERM technique. Chiang et al., (1981) observed pH range from 4.0 to 6.0 as optimum for fermentation of D-Xylulose to ethanol.

From the results on the effect of pH on ethanol production it may be concluded that a pH of 5.0 is optimum for fermentation of mango juice to ethanol.

2.5 KMS Concentration vs Ethanol Fermentation:

The results of the effect of different concentration of potassium metabisulphite (KMS) (50, 80, 100 and 125 ppm) on alcoholic fermentation of mango juice are presented in Table 6.

It has been observed that the rate of fermentation decreased considerably with the increase in KMS concentration. Fermentation completed within 96 hours with KMS concentration 50 ppm, whereas after the same fermentation period not even 50 percent of the substrate had been utilized with KMS concentration 125 ppm. Almost 50 percent of the substrate was utilized within 36, 60 and 72 hrs for treatment with KMS @ 50, 80 and 100 ppm respectively.

After 96 hrs of fermentation the TSS values observed for KMS treatments @ 50, 80, 100 and 125 ppm have been 2.4, 5.0, 7.2 and 13.0 respectively.

The amount of substrate utilized by yeast after 96 hrs of fermentation was found to be 88, 75, 64 and 35 percent with KMS concentration of 50, 80, 100 and 125 ppm respectively.

Table 6: KMS vs Alcoholic Fermentation

Fermentation period (hr)	KMS Concentration (ppm)			
	50	80	100	125
	TSS °Brix			
0	20.0	20.0	20.0	20.0
12	18.0	18.0	18.0	18.4
24	16.0	16.6	17.0	17.6
36	10.2	13.4	15.2	17.0
48	5.4	11.2	13.6	16.2
60	4.2	9.0	11.4	15.4
72	3.0	7.8	9.0	14.0
84	2.6	6.2	8.4	13.5
96	2.4	5.0	7.2	13.0

Fermentation Conditions:
    Initial TSS : 20.0 °B
    Inoculum @ : 15% (v/v)
    Temperature: 30 ± 2 °C
    pH : 5.0

From the above experiment conducted to see the effect of KMS on ethanol fermentation it may be concluded that KMS concentration @ 50 ppm has been optimum to prevent contamination of the fermenting mash.

Beech (1972) reported the use of SO_2 and asserted that it was necessary to add 75 pom of SO_2 in apple juice to check microbial population of the juice. White and Ough (1975) reported that 35 mg SO_2 per liter of juice is sufficient to inhibit the polyphenol oxidase enzyme completely. It may be concluded from the above that KMS (50 ppm) is optimum for the alcoholic fermentation of mango juice.

3. Optimum Fermentation Conditions:

The optimum fermentation conditions for the production of mango wine as concluded from the various optimization experiments are given in Table 7.

Table 7: Optimum conditions for production of mango wine

Total Soluble Solids (TSS, °Brix)	20.0
Organism	*Saccharomyces cerevisiae* var. ellipsoideus
Inoculum (% v/v)	15
pH	5.0
Fermentation temperature (°C)	30
Fermentation period (Hrs)	96
Potassium metabisulphite KMS (ppm)	50.0

4. Analysis and Evaluation of Mango Wine

The wine produced from mango juice supplemented with cane sugar has been chemically analyzed and evaluated and the results have been presented in Table 8.

Table 8: Analysis of Mango wine

Ethyl alcohol (% v/v)	9.0
Total Soluble Solids (°Brix)	2.4
Reducing sugars (g%)	0.08
Total acids (% tartaric acid)	0.40
Volatile acids (% Acetic acid)	0.001
pH	5.4
Grading	Commercially outstanding

5. Dehydration of Aqueous Ethanol for Fuel Alcohol

The wine produced from mango has been distilled at 68 ± 2 °C and distillate thus collected contained 95 percent ethanol. The distillate was dehydrated with calcium chloride @ 18 g/100 ml of distillate. The mixture was redistilled to collect dehydrated ethanol containing 99.5 per cent ethanol which may be used as a liquid fuel.

Chapter V - SUMMARY

The energy consumption in the world is increasing at an alarming rate and the non-renewable sources of energy are getting depleted rapidly. This acute energy problem has caused renewed interest in alternative and renewable sources of energy and fuel.

Mango (*Mangifera indica*) is the first most important fruit of Punjab state. It is grown on 11,022 hectares of land with an annual production of 66,132 tons. Out of this about 25-30% are wasted. The bulk of wastage of horticultural produce is mainly due to lack of proper facilities for transport, refrigerated storage and processing. In the present investigation substandard and waste mangoes (var. Dussehri) have been successfully utilized for the production of wines of outstanding quality and fuel alcohol. This will help to improve the economics of the fruit production and also prevent environmental pollution caused by decaying fruit.

The experiments were conducted to optimize various conditions for alcoholic fermentation of mango juice by *Saccharomyces cerevisiae* var. ellipsoideus. This yeast fermented mango juice efficiently at 30 ± 2 °C with inoculum concentration 15% (v/v). Out of the other conditions optimized 20.0 °Brix at pH 5.0 was recorded to be optimal for alcoholic fermentation. Potassium metabisulphite (KMS @ 50 ppm) prevented contamination. Fermentation of the mash from substandard fruits completed within 96 hours. Chemical analysis and sensory evaluation have classified the wine as of commercially out-standing quality.

Aqueous ethanol was dehydrated with calcium chloride (@ 18 gm/100 ml) yielding 99.5% ethyl alcohol which can be used as liquid fuel.

LITERATURE CITED

Abou Zeid, A. Z. A. and M. A. Farid. 1978. Fermentative production of ethyl alcohol by *Saccharomyces sp. Indian Chem. Manuf.* **16**(11):1.

Abou Zeid, M. M. and C. A. Reddy. 1986. Direct fermentation of potato starch to ethanol by co-cultures of *Aspergillus niger* and *S. cerevisiae*. *Appl. and Env. Micro.* **52**(5):1055-1059.

"Abou Zeid, M. M. and C.A. Reddy. 1987. Fermentation of starch to ethanol by a complementary mixture of an amylolytic yeast and *Saccharomyces cerevisiac. Biotechnol. Lett.* **9**(1):59-62.

Agrawal, P. and U. Veeramallu. 1990. Ethanol fermentation by *Zymomonas mobilis* ATCC 10988 in repeated batch cultures. *J. Chem. Technol. Biotechnol.* **47**(1):1-14.

Aires Barros, M.R., J.M.S. Cabral and J.M. Navais. 1987. Production of ethanol by immobilized *Saccharomyces bayanus* in an extractive fermentation system. *Biotechnol. Bioeng.* **29**(9):1097-1104.

Akpan, I., M.J. Tkenebomeh, N. Uraih and C.O. Obuckwe. 1988. Production of ethanol from cassava whey. *Acta Biotechnol.* **8**(1):39-45.

*Alian, A. and H. M. Musenge. 1970. Utilization of pineapple waste for wine making. *Zambia J. Sci. Technol.* **1**(1):29-33.

Amerine, M.A., H.W. Berg and W.V. Cruess. 1967. Technology of wine making. The AVI Publishing Co. Inc. Evaluation of wines and brandies: 678-724.

Amerine, M.A. and V.L.Singleton. 1968. Wine: An Introduction for Americans. University of California Press Berkeley and Los Angeles.

Amerine, M.A. and R.E.Kunkee. 1968. Microbiology of wine making. *Ann. Rev. Microbiol.* **22**:323-358.

Amerine, M.A., R.E. Kunkee, C.S. Ough, V.L. Singleton and A.D. Webb. 1980. The technology of wine making 4th ed., The AVI Publishing Co. Westport, C.T.

Amin, G. and H.W. Doelle. 1989, Vertical rotating immobilized cell reactor of the bacterium *Z. mobilis* for stable long-term continuous ethanol production. *Biotechnol. Tech.* **3**(2):95-100.

Angelino, S.A.G.F., H.C.M. Mocking-Bode and H.A. Vermeire. 1989. Activity of sulphate-metabolizing enzymes and sulphur dioxide formation during main fermentation. *Brauwissenschaft.* **42**(12):476-481.

Anshula. 1987. Studies on natural vinegar fermentation from *Syzuyium cuminii* M.Sc. Thesis: Punjab Agric. Univ., Ludhiana

Archer, D.B. and L.A. Thompson. 1987. Energy production through treatment of wastes by microorganisms: Changing perspectives in Applied Microbiology. C.S.Gutteridge and J.R.Norris (eds.), J. Appl. Bacteriol. **63**:596-705.

Association of Official Analytical Chemists. 1980. Official methods of analysis, A.O.A.C. 13th Ed. Washington, DC. 504

Avgerinos, G.C., H.Y. Fang, I. Biocic and DIC Wang. 1980. A novel single step microbiological conversion of cellulosic biomass to a liquid fuel ethanol, VI Int. Ferm. Symp and V. Int. Symp on Yeast, Canada. 1980:80.

Bacova, E., J. Kunider and J. Gawel. 1986. Technology of complex using of whey Prum. Potravin. **37**(4):209.

Baisya, RK. 1980. Fruits and vegetables processing industries in rural India—its problems and prospects. Indian Food Packer. **34**(6)29-32.

Bajpai, P., A. Sharma, N. Raghuram and P.K.Bajpai. 1988. Rapid production of ethanol in high concentration by immobilized cells of S. cerevisiae through soya flour supplementation. Biotechnol. Lett. **10**(3):217-220.

Bajpai, P., N. Verma and P.K Bajpai. 1989. Continuous ethanol production using immobilized cells of high-ethanol-producing yeast. Biotechnol. Appl Biochem. **11**(5):471-476.

Banerjee, B., J. Dasgupta, A.W. Khan, §.K.Basu, 8.D.Khandiya and V. Chandra.

1984. Fuel alcohol production from sugar beet and sweet sorghum, Indian J. Microbiol. 24(3-4):283-284.

Baronaik, A., B. Achremowicz and A. Wozniak. 1987. Continuous production of ethanol by immobilized yeast cells. *Acta Microbiol. Pol.* **36**(1-2):61.66,

Barrots, T.J., de Menezes. 1982. Starchy material for alcohol fuel production, Pro Biochem. **17**(3):32-34.

Beavan, M., B. Zawadzki, R. Droniuk, H. Lawford and J.Fein. 1989. Comparative performance trials with yeast and Zymomonas for fuel alcohol production from corn. 10th Symposium on Biotech. for Fuels and Chemicals, USA. Appl, Biochem. Biotechnol. **20-21**: 319-326.

Bechard, P., C. Jolicoeur and A. Beaubien. 1987. Toxicity effects of alcohols on Saccharomyces cerevisiae. A flow micro calorimetry investigation. Biotechnol. Tech. **1**(2):73-78.

Beech, F.W. 1972. English cider making technology, microbiology and biochemistry. Progress in Industrial Microbiology (**II**) :133-294. Churchill Livingstone Edinburg, London.

Bhanot, U.K. 1989. Fruit and Vegetable handling poor. Tribune 27th June: 3.

Borrego, F., J.M. Obon, M. Canovas, A. Manjon and J.L.Iborra. 1987. Effect of temperature and long-term operation on passively immobilized Z. mobilis for continuous ethanol production. Biotechnol. Lett. **9**(8):573-576.

Borrego, F., J.M.Obon, M. Canovas, A. Manjon and J.L.Tborra. 1988. pH influence on ethanol production and retained biomass in a passively immobilised Z. mobilis system. Biotechnol. Lett. **10**(6):437-442.

Bothast, R.J. and P.J. Slininger. 1984. Current development for immobilized living cells in continuous production of ethanol. V Canadian bioenergy R & D Seminar, Ottawa 1984.

Bowman, O.L. and E. Geiger. 1984. Optimization of fermentation conditions for alcohol production. Biotechnol. Bioeng. **26**(12):1492-1497.

Caputi, Jr. A. and D. Wright. 1969. Collaborative study of the determination of ethanol in wine by chemical oxidation. J. Assoc. of Anal. Chem. **52**(1):85.

Cason, D.T., G.C. Reid and E.M.S. Gatner. 1987. On the differing rates of fructose and glucose utilization in S. cerevisiae. J. Inst. Brew. **93**(1):23-25.

Cason, D.T., G.C. Reid and E.M.S. Gatner. 1987. Pitching rates related to glucose and fructose utilization in S. cerevisiae. J. Inst. Brew. **93**(6) 506-508.

Castellar, M.R., F. Borrego, M. Canovas, A. Manjon and J.L.Iborra. 1989. Continuous ethanol production at high glucose concentrations by a passively immobilised *Z. mobilis* system. Appl. Microbiol. Biotechnol. **31**(3):249-252.

Cheema, A. 1989 Production of ethanol from guava. M.Sc. Thesis. Punjab Agric. Univ. Ludhiana

Chen, H.C. and D.G.Mou. 1990. Pilot-scale multi-stage multi-feeding continuous ethanol fermentation using non-sterile cane molasses. Biotechnol. Lett. **12**(5):367-372.

Chiang, Lin-Chang, Cheng-Shung Gong, Li-fu Chen and George T. Tsao. 1981. D-Xylulose fermentation to ethanol by S. cerevisiae. Appl. Env. Microbiol. **42**(2):284.289.

Chithra, N. and A. Baradarajan. 1989. Studies on cd-immobilization of amyloglucosidase and S. cerevisiae for direct conversion of starch to ethanol. Process Biochem. **24**(6):208-211.

Cochet, N., M. Nonus and J.M.Lebeault. 1988. Solid-state fermentation of sugar-beet. Biotechnol. Lett. **10**(7):491-496.

Dallman, K., Z. Buzas and B. Szajani. 1987. Continuous fermentation of apple juice by immobilised yeast cells. Biotechnol. Lett. 9(8):577-580.

D'Amore, T., and G.G.Stewart. 1987. Ethanol tolerance of yeast. Enzyme Microb. Technol. **9**(6):322-330.

D'Amore, T., C.J. Panchal and G.G.Stewart. 1987. The effect of osmotic pressure on the intracellular accumulation of ethanol in S. cerevisiae during fermentation in wort. J. Inst. Brew. **93**(6):472-476.

D'Amore, T., C.J. Panchal, I. Russell and G.G.Stewart. 1988. Osmotic pressure effects and intracellular accumulation of ethanol in yeast during fermentation. J. Ind. Microbiol. **2**(6):365-372.

De Franca, F.P., D.S. Mano and S.G.F. Leite. 1986. Alcoholic fermentation of mandioc flour by *Zymomonas* sp. Rev. Latinoam. Microbiol. **28**(4):313-316.

*Deshpande, V., S. Keskar, C. Mishra and M. Rao. 1986. Direct conversion of cellulose /hemicellulose to ethanol by Neurospora crassa. Enzyme Microb. Technol. **8**(3):149-152.

Devine, S.I. and J.C. Slaughter. 1980. The effect of medium composition on the production of ethanol by S. cerevisiae. FEMS Microbiol. Lett.: **9**(1):19-21.

Dhawan,S.S., R.L.Kainsa and O.P. Gupta. 1983. Screening of guava cultivars for wine and brandy making. Haryana Agric. Univ. J. Res. **13**(3):420-423.

Doelle, M.B. and H.W.Doelle. 1989. Ethanol production from sugarcane syrup using Z. mobilis. J. Biotechnol. **11**(1):25-36.

Dombek, K.M. and L.O. Ingram. 1986. Magnesium Limitation and its role in apparent toxicity of ethanol during yeast fermentation. Appl. Environ. Microbiol. **52**(5):975-981.

Dombek,K.M. and L.O. Ingram. 1987. Ethanol production during batch fermentation with S. cerevisiae:Changes in glycolytic enzymes and internal PH. Appl. Environ. Microbiol. **53**(6):1286-1291.

Dyer, W.G. 1980. Methanol-Gasoline blends in New Zealand. Proc. of 4th Int. Symp. on alcohol Fuels technology. **2**:533-540.

Eurico da Fonseca. 1980. Alcohol fuels in Portugal. Proc. of 4th Int. Symp. On alcohol Fuels technology. **2**:843

*Fang, B.S., H.Y. Fang, C.S. Wu and C.T. Pan. 1984. High productivity ethanol production by immobilized yeast cells. Vth Symp. on Biotech. for Fuels and Chemicals. **1983**:457-464.

Faust, V. and P. Prave. 1980. An integral approach to power alcohol production. Proc. of 4th Int. Symp. on alcohol Fuels technology. 1:3-7.

Fleet, G.H. and Chong Xiao Gao. 1988. The effects of temperature and pH on the ethanol tolerance of the wine yeasts, S. cerevisiae, Candida stellata and Kloeckera apiculata. J. Appl. Bacteriol. **65**(5):405-409.

Fleet, G.H., G.M.Heard and C. Gao. 1989. The effect of temperature on growth and ethanol tolerance of yeasts during wine fermentation. 7th International Symposium on Yeasts, Perugia (Italy). Yeast. **2**:543-546.

Friend, B.A. and K.M. Shahan. 1981. Fuels from biomass and wastes. Publ. Ann. Arbor. Science Publishers; Inc. 343-355.

*Fukushima, S. and H. Hatakeyama. 1982. Novel immobilized bioreactor for rapid continuous ethanol fermentation of cane juice or fruit juices. IIIrd Biochemical Engineering Conf. Santa Barbara 1983. **413**:483-485.

Fumi, M.D., G.Trioli, M.G. Colombi and 0. Colagrande. 1988. Immobilization of S. cerevisiae in calcium alginate gel and its application to bottle fermented sparkling wine production. Am. J. Enol. Vitic. **39**(4):267-272.

Gadd, G.M. 1988. Carbon nutrition and metabolism. Pub. Blackwell Scientific Publications. Cambridge (USA) 1988:21-57(c.f. Microbiol. Abstr. A(1989) **24**(8):4987).

Gandhi, D.N. 1989. Production of some useful products of industrial importance through microbial fermentation of whey. Indian Dairyman. **41**(4):182-184.

Ghareib, M., K.A. Youssef and A.A.Khalil. 1988. Ethanol tolerance of S. cerevisiae and its relationship to lipid content and composition. Folia Microbiol. **33**(6):447-452.

Ghommidh, C. and J.D. Bu'lock. 1988. Ethanol production with artificially flocculated Zymomonas cells. Biotechnol. Tech. **2**(4):249-252.

Ghose, T.K. and R.D. Tyagi. 1979. Rapid ethanol fermentation of cellulose hydrolysate. 1. Batch vs continuous systems. Biotechnol. Bioeng. **21**:1387-1400.

Gibbons, W.R. and C.A. Westby. 1986. Use of Potassium metabisulfite to control bacterial contaminants during fermentation of fodder beet cubes for fuel ethanol. Biomass. **2**(2):99-113.

*Gong, C.8., L.F. Chen, M.C. Flickinger and G.T.Tsao. 1984. Production of ethanol by yeast using Xylulose. U.S. Patent. **4**:468-490.

Greenshield, R.N. 1975a. Malt vinegar manufacture. Brewer. **61**(729):295-298)[c.f. FSTA(1976)8:3T90]

Greenshield, R.N. 1975b. Malt vinegar manufacture. Brewer. **61**(732):401-407(c. FSTA(1976)8:5T196)

Greenshield, R.N. 1975. Octagen paper (2):20-27. University of Manchester, U.K.(c.f. A. Wiley Interscience Publication, N.Y. Ed. H.R. Bungay, 1980:347)

Grewal, H. S. 1986. Studies on vinegar fermentation from fruits. Ph.D Thesis. Punjab Agric. Univ. Ludhiana.

Grewal, H.S., H.K.Tewari and K.L.Kalra. 1988. Vinegar production from substandard fruits. Biological Wastes. **26**:9-14.

Grewal, H.S. and H.K.Tewari. 1990. Studies on vinegar production from plums. J. Res. Punjab. Agric. Univ. **26**(2):272-275.

"Grote, W. and P.L.Rogers. 1985. Ethanol production from sucrose based raw materials using immobilized cells of Zymomonas mobilis. Biomass. **8**(3):169-184.

Gupta, R.K. and J. S. Ahluwalia. 1980. Utilization of ethanol in Indian cars, scooters, motorcycles and tractors. Proc. of 4th Int. Symp. on alcohol Fuels technology.1980. **2**:543-550.

Haegerdal, H. B. and B. Mattiasson. 1982. Azide sterilization of fermentation media. Ethanol production from glucose using immobilized *S. cerevisiae*. Eur. J. Appl. Microbiol. Biotechnol. **14**(3):140-143.

Halos, S.C, M. Aussielita, L. Lit and W.T. Cruz. 1987. Effect of media sterilization and of varying sources and concentration of sugar and nitrogen on alcohol production by *S. cerevisiae* strains. Philipp. J. Sci. **116**(1)75 8.

Hang, Y.D., C.Y.Lee, E.F. Woodams and H.J.Cooley. 1981. Production of alcohol from fruit waste apple pomace. Appl. Env. Microbiol. **42**(6):1128-1129.

Hang, Y.D., C.Y. Lee and EF. Woodams. 1986. Solid state fermentation of grape pomace for ethanol production. Biotechnol. Lett. **8**(1):53.56,

Harris, J. R. Muider, D.B. Kell, R.P. Walter and J.G. Morris 1986. Solvent production of *Clostridium pasteurianum* in media of high sugar content. Biotechnol. Lett. **8**(12):889-892.

*Hartley, B.S. and G. Sharma 1987. Novel ethanol fermentation from sugarcane and pray. Utilization of lignocellulosic wastes. B.S. Hartley. bai x. Broda, P.J.Senior (eds.), 1987: 555-568,

*Heitland, H., H. Czaschke and N. Pinte. 1977. The case of alcohol from biomass 2s an alternative fuel in Brazil translation of conference, NTIS.

Hill, G.A. and C.W. Robinson. 1988. Morphological behavior of S. cerevisiae during continuous fermentation. Biotechnol, Lett. **10**(11):815-820.

Ho, Y.C. and H. M. Ghazali. 1986. Alcohol production from cassava starch by coimmobilised Z. mobilis and immobilised glucoamylase. Pertanika. **9**(2):235-240.

Hoshino, K., M. Taniguchi, H. Marumoto and M. Fujii. 1989. Repeated batch conversion of raw starch to ethanol using amylase immobilised on a reversible soluble-auto precipitating carrier and flocculating yeast cells. Agric. Biol. Chem. **53**(7):1961-1967.

Ingamells, J.C. and R.H Lindquist. 1975. Methanol as a motor fuel or a gasoline blending component. Proc. of 4th Int. Symp. on alcohol Fuels technology. Brazil. 1980. SAE paper No. 750123

Ingledew, W.M. and G.P.Casey. 1986. Rapid production of high concentrations of ethanol using unmodified industrial yeast. Biotechnol. and Renewable Energy: 246-257.

*Ingledew, W.W. and R.E. Kunkee. 1985. Factors influencing sluggish fermentations of grape juice. Am. J. Enol. Vitic. **36**(1) 165-76.

Ivanova, V., M.Rychtera and G.Basarova. 1989. The use of immobilised cells of yeast *Saccharomyces cerevisiae* for continuous ethanol production. I.Prospects of Applications. Kvasny Prum. **35**(2):41.44

Jayaraman, K.S. 1979. Dragging feet of gasohol. Science Today **13**(14):12.

Jimenez, J. and T. Benitex. 1987. Adaptation of yeast cell membranes to ethanol, Appl. Environ. Microbiol. **53**(5) :1196-1198

Jinescu, G., V.Lavric, S.Bragarea and M. Popescu. 1089. Mathematical modelling of immobilised living yeast cell reactor for sugar bioconversion to ethanol. Acta Biotechnol. **9**(4):325-332.

*Jirku, V. 1987. Ethanol tolerance of yeast cell. Kvansny Prum. **33**(4):106-108.

Jones, RP. and P.F. Greenfield. 1987, Specific and non-specific inhibitory effects of ethanol on yeast growth. Enzyme Microb. Technol. **9**(6):334-338.

Jones, R.P. 1988. Intracellular ethanol-accumulation and exit from yeast and other. cells. Fems. Microbiol. Rev. **54**(3):239. 258.

Kaeppeli, O and B. Sonnleitner. 1986. Regulation of sugar metabolism in Saccharomyces type yeast. Experimental ang conceptual considerations. CRC. CRIT Rev. Biotechnol. **4**(3): 299.356.

Kahlon, S.S. and P.Kumar. 1987. Simulation of fermentation conditions for ethanol production from water hyacinth. Indian J. Ecol. **14**(2):213-217.

*Karaki, I. 1974, Manufacture and use of industrial alcohol in Japan. Kagakh Kyoiku. **22**(5):365.

Khattak, J.N., M.K. Hamdy and J.J. Powers. 1965. Utilization of watermelon juice. 1. Alcoholic fermentation. Food Technol. **19**(8):1284-1286.

*King, D.W., T.M. Placzek, A. Duda and Sons. 1985. Process for manufacture of ethyl alcohol from citrus molasses. US patent 4,503,079. March 1985.

Klar. 1936. Fab. Abs. Alc. (cf. Alcohol--a Fuel for internal combustion engines, by S.J.W. Pleeth, 1949. Pub. Chapman and Hall Ltd., London)

*Klass, D.L. 1980. Alcohol fuels for motor vehicles. An over view, Energy Topics. 1980.

Klass, D.L. 1981. Fuels from biomass and wastes. Publ: Ann. Arbor. Science Publishers; Inc.: 1-38.

Kunhi, A.A.M, N.D. Ghildyal, B.K. Lonsane, S.Y. Ahmed and C.P. Nataranjan. 1980. Studies on production of alcohol from saccharified waste residue from cassava. Starch processing industry. Starch. **33**(8):275-279.

*Klyosov, A.A. 1985. Enzymatic conversion of cellulose to sugars and alcohol: Present state of the art. Prinkl. Biokhim. Mikrobiol. **21**(2): 269-283.

Klyosov, A.A. 1986. Enzymatic conversion of cellulosic materials to sugar and alcohol: The technology and its implication. Appl. Biochem. Biotechnol. **12**(3): 249-300.

Lafourcade, L. S. 1983. Wine and Brandy. Biotechnology. Edited by H.J.Rehm and G. Reed. **5**:81-163.

*Laude-Bousget, A. 1989. Process and apparatus for thermal control of winemaking. US Patent. 4,814,189. March, 1989.

"Lawford, H.G. 1988. Ethanol production by high performance bacterial fermentation. US Patent. 4,731,329. March, 1988.

Lawford, H., P. Holloway and A. Ruggiero, 1988. Effect of pH on growth and ethanol production by *Zymononas*. Biotechnol. Lett. **10**(11): 809-814.

*Lawford, H.G. 1989. Ethanol production by high performance bacterial fermentation. US Patent 4,830,964. May, 1989.

*Lawford, H.G. 1989. Continuous process for ethanol production by bacterial fermentation. US Patent. 4,816,399. March, 1989.

Lawford, H. G. and A. Ruggiero. 1990. Production of fuel alcohol by Zymomonas: Effect of pH on maintenance and growth-associated metabolism. Biotechnol Appl. Biochem. **12**(2): 206-211.

Lee, J.H, D.Williamson and P.L.C.Sch. Roger. 1980. The effect of temperature on kinetics of ethanol production by *S.cerevisiae*. Biotechnol. Loti. 2.141

*Lee, C.Y. and R.W. Kime. 1990. Stabilization of wine with honey and sulphur dioxide. US Patent. 4,900,564. Feb., 1990.

Leite, S.G.F and F.P. Franca. 1988. Preliminary study of the effect of the addition of ethanol to the alcoholic fermentation carried out by *S. cerevisiae*. Rev. Microbiol. **19**(4): 430-431.

*Lembke, A.E. Uderberg and H.J. Strobel. 1990. Process for the production of sparkling wine. US Patent. 4,948,598. Aug., 1990.

Lokendra Singh. 1984. Production of ethyl alcohol from agricultural cellulosic wastes. Ph.D. Thesis. Punjab Agric. Univ. Ludhiana.

*Maeda, HY. Kimura and S Kajiwara. 1985. Immobilization of yeast cells and the continuous ethanol production. Rep. Ferment. Res. Inst. **64**:19.24

Mann, E.J. 1980. Alcohol from whey. Dairy Ind. Int. **45**(3): 47-48,

Maiorella, B.L. 1085. Ethanol comprehensive. Biotech. **3**: 861-914, Ed: M. Moo-young. Pergamon Press U.S.A.

Maldonado, O., C.Rolz and S. Schneider de/Cabrera. 1975. Wine and vinegar production from tropical fruits. J. Food, Soi **40**:262-265.

*Matsumoto, I. and T. Yamamoto. 1973. Oxyfuels.1. Properties of gasoline containing alcohols. Nenryo kyokaishi. **52**(8): 680.

Marwaha, S.S., J.F. Kennedy and H.K.Tewari. 1985. A review-Immobilization of yeasts. Proc. National Symp. Yeast Biotech. Haryana Agric. Univ. : 76.95.
Marwaha, S.S., J.F. Kennedy and H.K. Tewari. 1986. A review-Role of immobilized whole cells in whey permeate treatment. Annals of Biology, 2(2): 203.214.
Marwaha, S.S., J.F.Kennedy, H.K.Tewari and A.Redhu. 1989, Characterization and treatment of dairy effluents by free and immobilised yeast. Process Biochem. : 46-51.
Marwaha, S.., J.F.Kennedy, P.K. Khanna, HK Tewari and A.Redhu 1990. Comparative investigations on the physiological parameters of free and immobilized yeast cells for effective treatment of dairy effluents. Proc. Int. Symp., Physiology of immobilised cells. Netherland. Elsevier Science Publishers, Amsterdam: 265-273.

*Menezes, T.O.B and P.R. Lomo. 1976. Production of alcohol from cassava. Boletin do Institute de Technologia de alimentos. Brazil, **46**: 37.54.

Menrad, H. 1977. Recent progress in automotive alcohol fuel application. Proc. Of IVth Int. Symp. on Automotive Propulsion systems, 1977:18-22,

Menrad,H.K., and H.Loeck. 1980. Results from basic research on alcohol powered vehicles. Proc. of IVth Int. Symp. on alcohol fuels technology. **2**: 557-562.

Miller,G.L. 1959. Use of dinitro salicylic acid reagent for determination of reducing sugars. Anal. Chem. **31**:426.428.

Miller,D.L. 1975. Ethanol fermentation and potential Biotechnol. Bioeng. Symp. **5**:345.

Miller, J.E., P.S. Weathers, F.X. Mc Conville and M. Goldberg. 1982 Saccharification and ethanol fermentation of apple pomace. 1V th Symposium, Biotechnology in Energy Production and Conservation Biotechnol. Bioeng. Symp. **12**:183-191.

Millichip, R.J. 1988. Ethanal production by Zymomonas cultures in yeast-conditioned media. US patent 4,885,241. Dec. 1980

*Minarik, E. 1985. Some microbiological and biotechnological problems in wine making. Kvasny Prum. **31**(7-8):182-183.

Morgan, E., G.Fleming, T. Patching and E. Colleran. 1989. Solid-state fermentation of sugar-beet for the purpose of fuel-alcohol production. Trans. Biochem.Soc. **17**(2):424.

*Mota, M. 1986. Production of fuel alcohols by fermentation physiological basis for improving the process. Presented at 1 contractor's Meeting, Brussels. 1986.

Mullins, J.T. and C.C.NeSmith. 1987. Acceleration of rate of ethanol fermentation by addition of nitrogen in high tannin grain sorghum. Biotechnol. Bioeng. **30**(9):1073-1076.

Nagashima, M., M. Azuma, S.Noguchi, K.Inuzuka and H. Samejima. 1984. Continuous ethanol fermentation using immobilized yeast cells Biotechnol. Bioeng. **26**(8): 992.997.

Nain, L.R and R.S. Rana. 1988. Ethanol production from sugar beet juice by S. Cerevisiae. Nutrient optimization studies. J. Maharashtra Agric. Univ. **13**(2): 141-144.

Nakamura, K., Y. Amano and O. Nakayama, 1989. Determination of free sulphite in Wine using a microbial sensor. Appl. Microbiol. Biotechnol. **31**(4):351-354.

Navarro, AR., M.C. Rubio and D.A.S. Callieri, 1983 Production of ethanol by yeasts immobilized in pectin. Eur. J. Appl. Microbiol, Biotechnol. **17**(3):148-151,

Neelam, 1987. Production of quality vinegar from Tow grade pears. M.Sc. Thesis. Punjab Agric. University. Ludhiana.

Ngang, J.O.E, F. Letourneau and P. Villa, 1989, Alcoholic fermentation of beet molasses: Effects of lactic acid on yeast fermentation parameters. Appl. Microbiol. Biotechnol. **31**(2):125-128.

Nunez, M.J. and J.M. Lema. 1987. Cell immobilization: Application to alcohol production. Enzyme Microb. Technol. **9**(11):642-651.

Obisanya, M.O., J.O. Aina and G.B.Oguntimein. 1987. Production of wine from mango using Saccharomyces and Schizosaccharomyces species isolated from palm wine. J. Appl. Bacteriol. **63**(3):191-196.

*Orlowski, J. and J. Barford. 1987. The effect of inoculum preparation on the fully aerated growth of S. cerevisiae with a glucose substrate. J.Gen. Appl.Microbiol. **33**:113-121.

Ough, C.8. and E.A. Crowell. 1987. Use of sulfur dioxide in wine making. J. Food Sci. **52**(2): 386-390.

Pampulha, M.E. and V. Loureiro. 1989. Interaction of the effects of acetic acid and ethanol on inhibition of fermentation in S. cerevisiae. Biotechnol. Lett. **11**(4):269-274.

Pampulha, M.E. and M.C.Loureior-Dias. 1989. Combined effect of acetic acid, pH and ethanol on intracellular pH of fermenting yeast. Appl. Microbiol. Biotechnol. **31**(5-6):547-550.

Panchal,P.J and G.G Stewart. 1980. The effect of osmotic pressure on the production and excretion of ethanol and glycerol by a brewing yeast strain. J. Inst. Brew. **86**:207-210

Panchal, C.T., C.A. Bilinski, I. Russel and G. Stewart. 1986. Yeast stability in the brewing and industrial fermentation ethanol industries CRC.Crit. Rev. Biotechnol. **4**(3): 263-298.

Parsons, R.V., N.G. Mc Duffle and G.A. Din 1984. pH inhibition of yeast ethanol fermentation in continuous culture. Biotechnol Lett. **16**(10): 677-680.

Pasari, A.B., R.A. Korus and R.C. Heimsch. 1989. A model for continuous fermentations with amylolytic yeasts. Biotechnol. Bioeng. **33**(3):338-343.

Passarinho, P.C.L.V., A.M.S. Vieira, J.M.S. Cabral, J.M. Novais and J.F. Kennedy. 1989. Effect of carrier matrix on fermentative production of ethanol by surface immobilised yeast cells. J. Chem. Technol. Biotechnol. **44**(3):183-194.

Patil, S.G. and B.G. Patil. 1989. Chitin supplement speeds up the ethanol production in cane molasses fermentation. Enzyme Microb. Technol. **11**(1):38-43.

Patil, S.G., D.V. Gokhale and B.G. Patil. 1989. Novel supplements enhance the ethanol production in cane molasses fermentation by recycling yeast cells. Biotechnol. Lett. **11**(3):213-216.

Patil, S.G. and B.G. Patil. 1989. Top and bottom yeasts together accelerate ethanol production in molasses fermentation. Biotechnol. Lett. **11**(5):359-364.

Pilando, L.S, R.E. Wrolstad and D.A. Heatherbell. 1985. Influence of fruit composition, maturity and mold contamination on the color and appearance of strawberry wine. J. Food. Sci. **50**(4) : 1121-1123.

Pleeth, S.J.W. 1949. Alcohol - a fuel for internal combustion engines. Chapman and Hall, London. 1949:259.

Pontiveros, C.R., J.A. Akontara and E.J. Rosodro. 1978, Acid saccharification and alcohol fermentation of unripe banana fruit. Philippine J. of Corp. Sei. **3**(3): 153-158.

Prouty, J.L., Davy Me Kee Corporation. 1980. The impact of differing raw materials and alternate fermentation methods on process designs for the production of fuel grade ethanol. Proc. of the IVth Int. Symp. on alcohol Fuels technology. **1**: 57-61

Prescott, S.C. and C.G. Dunn 1949. Industrial Microbiology. 4th ed. Mc Graw-hill Book Co., New York.

Pundle, A., A. Prabhune and H. Sivaraman. 1988. Immobilization of *S.uvarum* cells in porous beads of polyacrylamide gel for ethanolic fermentation. Appl. Microbiol. Biotechnol. **29**(5):426-429.

Ramos, M.T. and A. Madeira-Lopes. 1990. Effects of acetic acid on the temperature profile of ethanol tolerance in S. cerevisiae. Biotechnol. Lett. **12**(3):229.234

Rao, G. and R. Mutharasan. 1986. Alcohol production by Clostridium acetobutylicum induced by methyl viologen. Biotechnol. Lett. **8**(12):893-896.

Rao, BS., A.V. Pundle, A.A. Prabhune, V.Shankar and H.Sivaraman. 1986, Ethanol production by yeast cells immobilized in open-pore agar. Appl. Biochem. Biotechnol. **21**(1): 17-24.

Reed, G. and T.W.Nagodawithana. 1988. Technology of yeast usage in winemaking. Am. J. Enol. Vitic. **39**(1):83-90.

Retamal, N., J.M. Duran and J. Fernandez. 1987. Ethanol production by fermentation of fruits and cladodes of prickly pear cactus. J. Sei, Food Agric. **40**(3):213-218.

Riboreau-Gayon, P. 1984. Relationship between the inhibition of alcoholic fermentation by S.cerevisiae. Biotechnol. Lett. **6**(10): 687-692.

Richter, K. and U Becker. 1985. Appearance of inhibition in the ethanol fermentation. IL. Influence of substrate concentration on the specific rate of ethanol production of S.cerevisiae. Acta Biotechnol. **5**(2): 145.152.

Richter, K. 1986. Inhibitory effects of ethanol in alcoholic fermentation Acta Biotechnol. **6**(3):237-243.

Richter, K. and U.Becker. 1987. Effects of temperature on microbial ethanol production.1. The temperature profile curve of ethanol production of the yeast strain S.cerevisiae Sc 5. Acta Biotechnol. **7**(1): 87-92.

Richter, K.1987. Effect of temperature on microbial ethanol production. II. A thermodynamic interpretation of the temperature profile curve of ethanol production. Acta Biotechnol. **7**(2): 127-140.

Richter, K., I. Ruchlemann and R. Berger. 1990. Ethanolic fermentation with S. cerevisiae cells immobilised in pectate gel. Acta Biotechnol. **10**(1):55.61.

Roberts, R.R. 1980. Alcohol production from molasses. Selection of efficient yeast strains. Energy Res. Abstr. **5**(13) (Abst.No. 20921)

Rodriguez, E. and D.A.S Callieri. 1986. High yield conversion of sucrose into ethanol by a flocculent Zymomonas sp. isolated from sugar cane juice. Biotechnol. Lett. **8**(10): 745-748.

Rogosa, M., HLH. Browne and E.O Wittier. 1947. Ethyl alcohol from Whey. J. Dairy Science. **30**(4): 263-269.

Rolz, C, S. de Cabrera and R. Garcia. 1980. Ethanol from sugar cane. The Ex-FERM Concept. Biotechnol. Bioeng. **21**:2347-2349.

Rosario, E.J. and F.V. Pamatong. 1985. Continuous flow fermentation of banana fruit pulp sugar into ethanol by carrageenan-immobilized yeast. Biotechnol. Lett. **7**(11): 819-820.

Sahm, H. and St. Bringer-Meyer. 1987. Continuous ethanol production by Z. mobilis on an industrial scale. Acta Biotechnol. **7**(4):307-313.

*Saida, T. 1989. Process for producing ethanol by fermentation. US Patent 4,822,737. April 1989.

*Salzbrunn, W., E. Steiner, W. Woehrer and O. Meixner. 1989. Method of continuously producing ethanol from sugar-containing substrates. US Patent 4,876,196. Oct. 1989.

Shamala, TR. and K.R.Sreekantiah. 1988. Use of wheat bran as a nutritive supplement for the production of ethanol by Z. mobilis. J. Appl. Bacteriol. **65**(6):433-436.

Shanker, V. , S.M.Kotwal and B.Scetarama Rao. 1985. Yeast cells entrapped in low gelling temperature agarose for the continuous production of ethanol. Biotechnol. Lett. **7**(8): 615-618.

Shih-Yow Huang, Jyh-Chern Chen. 1988. Analysis of kinetics of ethanol fermentation with Z. mobilis considering temperature effect. Enzyme Microb. Technol. **10**(7):431-439.

Sivaraman, H., B.S. Rao and A.V. Pundle. 1982. Continuous ethanol production by yeast cells immobilized in open pore gelatin matrix. Biotechnol. Lett, 496):359-364.

Sreekantiah, K.R., Satyanaryana and B.A. Rao. 1980. Production of ethanol from tubers. J. Food. Sci. Technol. **17**(4):194-195.

*Stone, J. 1974. Survey of alcohol fuel technology. An interim report to Mitre corp. Mclean. Virginia.

Stein, M.A.C.F. 1986. Banana wine. Cienc. Cult. **38**(2): 362-366.

Strehaiano, P. M. Mota and G. Goma. 1983. Effect of inoculum level on kinetics of alcohol fermentation. Biotechnol. Lett. **5**(2): 135-140.

Tangnu, S.K. 1982. Process development for ethanol production based on enzymatic hydrolysis of cellulosic biomass. Process Biochem. **17**(3): 36.45.

*Tedder,D.W. 1985. Process for producing fuel grade ethanol by continuous fermentation, solvent extraction and alcohol separation Georgia Tech Research Corp. Atlanta, US Patent 4, 517, 298.

Tewari H.K. 1978. Prospectus of somras making at home, Proc Production of Somras. Punjab. Agric. Univ. 1:22.28.
Tewari H.K., R.P.Sethi and D.S.Chahal. 1978. Screening of grape varieties on the Punjab State for their enological qualities. Proc. Industrial Fermentation Symp. Jammu (J & K), India.
Tewari,H.K. and L.K.Gupta. 1978. Somras as food and medicines, Proc. Production of Somras. Punjab Agric. Univ. **1**:29-40.
Tewari, HK. 1978. Feasibility report on grapes and their Processing in Punjab State.
Tewari, H.K. 1978. Report on the establishment of experimental winery, MARKFED, Chandigarh.
Tewari, HK. 1978. Report on the establishment of pilot scale grape processing plant for wines and brandy.
Tewari, HK and S, K. Ghai. 1978. Grape culture and somras production. Proc. Production of

Somras. Punjab Agric. Univ, **1**:8-21.
Tewari,H.K. 1979. Karele da Somras. Yuvrishma, Punjab Agric. Univ. **6**(4):21-22.
Tewari, H.K. 1979. Somras. Yuvrishma. Punjab Agric. Univ **6**(2-3):19.
Tewari, H.K. 1979. A manual for diabetics. Punjab Agric. Univ. Ludhiana.
Tewari, HK. 1980. Somras our Vedic drink. Proc. Assoc. Food Science and Tech. Ludhiana. **3**:15-16.
Tewari,H.K. 1980. Karele da Somras. Package Samachar, Agric. Deptt. Punjab State:2-4.
Tewari,H.K. 1981. Remedy for Madhumeha - Diabetes. Vigyan Pragati. **2**:186.
Tewari, HK., L.Singh and R.P.Sethi. 1982. Isolation of yeast strains from fruits for bioconversion of waste potato to ethanol. Proc. 1st National Symp. Biotech. Chandigarh: 284-291.
Tewari, HK, L. Singh and R.P Sethi. 1982, Utilization of waste potato for the production of ethanol. Punjab Horticultural J. **22**(3-4): 914.214
Tewari, H.K., L.Singh and R.P.Sethi. 1983. Production of alcohol from potato. J. Res. Punjab Agric. Univ. **20**(1):74-80.
Tewari, H.K., S.S. Marwaha and N. Sehgal. 1985. Studies on active dry wine yeast tablets. Proc. National Symp. Yeast Biotechnology, Haryana Agric. Univ. Hisar. 1985:153-159.
Tewari, H.K., S.S. Marwaha and L. Singh. 1985. Ethanol production from acid and enzymatic hydrolysates of saw dust. Ann. Biol. India **1**(27):215-222.
Tewari, H.K., S.S. Marwaha and K. Rupal. 1986. Ethanol from banana peels. Agric. Wastes. **16**(2):135-146.
Tewari, HK, S.8. Marwaha, K. Rupal and L. Singh. 1986. Production of ethyl alcohol from banana peels. J. Res. Punjab Agric. Univ, **22**(4): 703-711.
Tewari,H.K. 1986. Karelian da Somras (wine) Kiwen Banayey. Changi Kheti. Punjab Agric. Univ. **22**(12):20-21.
Tewari,H.K., S.S. Marwaha, J.F. Kennedy and L. Singh. 1987. Acid and enzymatic saccharification of agricultural mixed polymers for alcohol production. British Polymer Journal. **19**:425.428.
Tewari,H.K., S.S. Marwaha, J.F. Kennedy and L. Singh. 1987. Role of pretreatments of enzymatic hydrolysis of agricultural residues for reducing sugar production. J Chem. Tech. Biotechnol. **38**:153-165.
Tewari,H.K., S.S. Marwaha, and N. Verma. 1987. Utilization of substandard pears for the production of wines and vinegar as food and medicine. Punjab Pear fruit Seminar. Punjab Agricultural University, Ludhiana.
Tewari,H.K., S.S. Marwaha, J.F. Kennedy and K. Rupal, 1987 Bio utilization of pineapple waste for ethanol generation. Wood and Celluloses, Industrial Utilization, Biotechnology, structure and properties. Pub-Ellis Horwood Ltd. and John Wiley U.K, U.S.A. and Canada. Chapter **27**: 251-259.
Tewari, H.K., S.S. Marwaha, J.F. Kennedy and L. Singh 1988, Evaluation of acids and cellulose enzyme for the effective hydrolysis of agricultural lignocellulosic residues. J. Chem Tech. Biotechnol. **41**: 261-275.
Tewari, H.K., H.S.Grewal and K.L Kalra, 1988. Vinegar production from substandard fruits. Biological Wastes. **26**:9-14.
Tewari,H.K., H.5.Grewal, S.S. Marwaha and Rakesh Sharma, 1988. Studies on the suitability of *Prunus salicina* (plum) for vinegar fermentation. Indigenous Medicinal Plants Symp: 1-14. Today and Tomorrow's Printers and Publishers, New Delhi.
Tewari, H.K., S.S. Marwaha and L. Singh. 1988. Studies on the screening of yeasts for ethanol production and treatment of dairy industry waste waters J. Res. Punjab Agric. Univ. **25**(1):81-87.

Tewari, H.K., S.S Marwaha, J.F. Kennedy and K. Rupal. 1989. Bioethanol generation from bio-polymers of vegetable wastes. Int. Ind. Biotechnol. **9**(5):15-19.

*Thorsson, C. 1989. Process for the production of ethanol through molasses fermentation. U.S Patent 4,886,751. December, 1989. (c.f. Microbiol. Abstr. A.(1990) **25**(9):5674).

*Toda, K., T.Asakura and H. Ohtake. 1987. Inhibitory effect of ethanol on ethanol fermentation. J. Gen. Appl. Microbiol. **33**(5):421-428.

Underkofler, L.A. and R.J. Hickey. 1954. Industrial fermentation. Chemical Publ. Co., New York. **1**:17.

Tuite, J. 1969. Plant Pathological Methods- fungi and bacteria. Burgess Publ, Co, Minneapolis Minn, U.S.A: 239.

Van Uden, N. 1984. Effects of ethanol on the temperature relations of viability growth in yeast. CRC.Crit. Rev. Biotechnol. **1**(3): 263-273.

Van Dijken, J.P. and W.A. Scheffer. 1984. Studies on alcoholic fermentation in yeasts. Innovations in Biotechnology. Prog. Ind. Microbiol. **120**:497-506.

Venugopal, B., S.M. Ibrahim and N.R. Kuloor. 1964. Dehydration of rectified spirit to absolute alcohol by solid desiccants. Chem. Age. India **15**(12):1255.

Viegas, C.A., M.F. Rosa, I. Sa-Correia and J.M. Novais. 1989. Inhibition of yeast growth by octanoic and decanoic acids produced during ethanolic fermentation. Appl. Environ. Microbiol. **55**(1):21-28.

Vyas, KK and V.K.Joshi, 1982. Plum wine making. Standardization of methodology. Indian Fd. Packer. **36**(6): 80-86.

Walker-Caprioglio, H.M and L.W. Parks. 1987. Auto conditioning factor relieves ethanol induced growth inhibition of S.cerevisiae. Appl. Environ, Microbial **53**(1):33-35.

*White, B.B and C.S. Ough. 1975. Oxygen uptake studies on grape juice. Am. J. Enol Vitic. **24**:184.

Yamamura, M., Y. Nagami, V. Vongsuvanlert, J. Kamnuanta and T. Kamihara. 1988. Effects of elevated temperature on growth, respiratory deficient mutation, respiratory activity and ethanol production in yeast. Can. J. Microbiol. /J. Can. Microbiol. **34**(8):1014-1017.

Zakrezewski, E. and S. Zmarlicki. 1988. Ethanolic fermentation in whey and whey molasses mixtures. II. Two-stage fermentation process of ethanol production from whey and beet molasses. Milchwissenschaft. **43**(8):492-496.

Zertuche, L and R.R. Zall. 1982. Production of ethanol from cellulose using *Clostridium thermocellum*. J. Fd. Sci. **47**(1): 328.

Original not seen.

Appendix I

Appendix I
Districtwise Area and Production of different fruits in the state as on 31.3.90

District\Fruits	A/P	Kinnow and other mandarins	Sweet orange	Lime lemon	Mango	Litchi	Guava	Pear	Peach	Plum	Grapes	Ber	Misc.	Total
Amritsar	A	1529	62	17	511	68	427	3058	555	63	5	19	102	6417
Amritsar	P	15290	310	85	3066	408	4270	45885	2325	252	135	76	285	78357
Bathinda	A	1369	457	67	64		153	68	54	2	1050	209	92	3589
Bathinda	P	13690	2335	305	384		1530	1020	810	8	28350	836	230	49498
Faridkot	A	2759	3863	74	71	3	134	173	161	8	221	95	346	8008
Faridkot	P	27390	19315	370	426	18	1340	4095	2415	32	5967	380	865	62813
Ferozepur	A	4030	5401	50	20		48	76	124	29	289	69	664	10800
Ferozepur	P	40300	27055	250	120		480	1140	1860	116	7803	276	1600	81010
Gurdaspur	A	1360	76	71	2543	834	282	300	204	99	9	2	984	6764
Gurdaspur	P	13600	380	355	15258	5004	2820	4500	3060	396	243	8	2460	48084
Hoshiarpur	A	3781	112	97	3767	167	459	352	377	58	1	31	265	9447
Hoshiarpur	P	37810	560	485	22602	1002	4590	5280	5655	152	27	124	663	78950
Jalandhar	A	1327	21	70	307	70	327	1496	388	67	42	31	108	4254
Jalandhar	P	13270	105	350	1842	420	3270	22440	5820	268	1134	124	270	49313
Kapur-thala	A	601	45	33	153	6	176	348	97	2	20	8	17	1506
Kapur-thala	P	6010	225	165	918	36	1760	5220	1455	8	540	32	42	16411
Ludhiana	A	942	42	221	578	5	511	421	271	5	193	235	419	3843
Ludhiana	P	9420	210	1103	3460	30	5110	6315	4065	20	5211	940	1048	36942
Patiala	A	1069	85	169	963	44	635	494	386	15	47	250	88	4245
Patiala	P	10690	425	845	5778	264	6350	7410	5790	60	1269	1000	220	40101
Ropar	A	785	48	171	1982	62	543	162	107	1	24	61	46	3992
Ropar	P	7850	240	855	11892	372	5430	2430	1605	4	648	244	115	31685
Sangrur	A	646	84	32	63	1	214	117	156		189	548	51	2082
Sangrur	P	6460	420	160	378	6	2140	1755	2040		5103	2196	127	20785
Total	A	20198	10306	1066	11022	1260	3909	7166	2860	329	2090	1559	3182	64947
Total	P	201980	51330	5330	66132	7560	39090	107490	42900	1316	56430	6236	7955	593949

A = Area in Hectares   P = Production in tons

Source: Directorate of Horticulture, Punjab

Publisher's Addendum

Publisher's Note

Latin terms and Scientific terms are printed in *italics*.
Author name prior marriage **Nandita Paul** at the time of writing the thesis, and post marriage **Nandita Gupta** presently.

Scans of Original (some)

Sample scanned pages from Original for sake of authenticity.

CERTIFICATE I

This is to certify that this thesis entitled "Studies on Wines and Fuel Alcohol Production" submitted for the degree of Master of Science in the subject of Microbiology [Minor Field : Food Science and Technology] of the Punjab Agricultural University, is a bonafide research work carried out by Nandita Paul (L-89-BS-100-M) under my supervision and that no part of this thesis has been submitted for any other degree.

The assistance and help received during the course of investigation have been fully acknowledged.

[Dr. H. K. Tewari]
Major Advisor
Mycologist
Deptt. of Microbiology

CERTIFICATE II

This is to certify that the thesis entitled "Studies on Wines and Fuel Alcohol Production" submitted by Nandita Paul (L-89-BS-100-M) to the Punjab Agricultural University in partial fulfilment of the requirements for the degree of Master of Science in the subject of Microbiology [Minor field: Food Science and Technology] has been approved by the Student's Advisory Committee after an oral examination on the same, in collaboration with an external examiner.

(Dr. H. K. Tewari)
Major Advisor

(Dr. R. S. Kahlon)
Head of the Department

(External Examiner)
Dr. S.S. MARWAHA
HEAD,
DEPT. OF BIOTECHNOLOGY,
PUNJABI UNIVERSITY,
PATIALA.

(Dr. D. S. Sidhu) 5 MAR 1992
Dean, Post-graduate Studies

Acknowledgements (part portion)

I am at a loss for words to express my deep sense of gratitude for my respected parents for their hearty blessings and ever encouraging moral support. I am also indebted to my loving brother, Ashwini and sister, Sangeeta, who have always stood by me and been a source of my strength.

Financial assistance in the form of merit fellowship given by Punjab Agricultural University, Ludhiana, during the tenure of my M.Sc. is gratefully acknowledged.

Dated: 30|12|91

Nandita Paul
[Nandita Paul]

ABSTRACT

Substandard and waste mango (*Mangifera indica*) var. Dussehri was utilised for ethanol fermentation by *Saccharomyces cerevisiae* var. ellipsoideus strain montrachet (@ 15% v/v). Ethanol 9.0% v/v was produced from the substrate with initial TSS of 20.0° B (pH 5.0). The optimum fermentation period was 96 hours at 30°C. Potassium metabisulphite (KMS @ 50 ppm) prevented contamination. Chemical analysis and sensory evaluation have classified the mango wine as of commercially outstanding quality. Aqueous ethanol was dehydrated with Calcium chloride (@18 gm/100 ml) yielding 99.5% ethyl alcohol which can be used as liquid fuel.

[Dr. H.K. Tewari] [Nandita Paul]

Contents

Chapter		Pages
I	INTRODUCTION	1-3
II	REVIEW OF LITERATURE	4-22
III	MATERIAL AND METHODS	23-32
IV	RESULTS AND DISCUSSION	33-48
V	SUMMARY	49-50
	LITERATURE CITED	i-xv
	APPENDIX	I

References

A list of some online References.

H. K. Tewari
https://in.linkedin.com/in/dr-harmesh-tewari-b4157a9

Parsons et al., 1987
https://www.sciencedirect.com/science/article/pii/B9780080331744500147

Bechard et al., 1987
https://link.springer.com/article/10.1007/BF00159325

D'Amore et al., 1987
https://www.sciencedirect.com/science/article/abs/pii/0141022987900536

Toda et al., 1987
https://www.jstage.jst.go.jp/article/jgam1955/33/5/33_5_421/_pdf/-char/ja

Ramos and Madeira-Lopes 1990
https://link.springer.com/article/10.1007/BF01026805

Jones and Greenfield 1987
https://espace.library.uq.edu.au/view/UQ:407514

Tedder 1985
https://patents.google.com/patent/US4517298

Shankar *et al.*, 1985
https://link.springer.com/article/10.1007/BF01026460

Hill and Robinson 1988
https://link.springer.com/article/10.1007/BF01027579

Mitchell *et al.*, 1988
https://link.springer.com/article/10.1007/BF01874199

Pasari *et al.*, 1989
https://pubmed.ncbi.nlm.nih.gov/18587922/

Grote and Rogers 1985
https://www.sciencedirect.com/science/article/abs/pii/0144456585900459

Deshpande *et al.*, 1986
https://www.sciencedirect.com/science/article/abs/pii/0141022986901031?via%3Dihub

Rao and Mutharasan 1986
https://link.springer.com/article/10.1007/BF01078655

Castellar *et al.*, 1989
https://link.springer.com/article/10.1007/BF00258404

Agrawal and Veeramallu 1990
https://onlinelibrary.wiley.com/doi/abs/10.1002/jctb.280470102

Obisanya *et al.*, 1987
https://ami-journals.onlinelibrary.wiley.com/doi/abs/10.1111/j.1365-2672.1987.tb04935.x

Laude *et al.*, 1987
https://patents.google.com/patent/EP0251944A1/en

Lee and Kime 1990
https://patents.google.com/patent/US4900564A/en

Lembke *et al.*, 1989
https://patents.google.com/patent/CA1304707C/no

Nagashima *et al.*, 1984
https://onlinelibrary.wiley.com/doi/abs/10.1002/bit.260260826

Hoshino *et al.*, 1989
https://www.tandfonline.com/doi/pdf/10.1080/00021369.1989.10869593

Epilogue

Life is Precious. Live every moment in Gratefulness, Kindness, Cheerfulness, Joy.

-

IT IS NOT EASY WITHOUT A MASTER.

सर्वे भवन्तु सुखिनः । सर्वे सन्तु निरामयाः ।

सर्वे भद्राणि पश्यन्तु । मा कश्चिद् दुःख भाग्भवेत् ॥

ॐ शान्तिः शान्तिः शान्तिः ॥

When faith has blossomed in life,
Every step is led by the Divine.

Sri Sri Ravi Shankar

Om Namah Shivaya

जय गुरुदेव

www.ingramcontent.com/pod-product-compliance
Lightning Source LLC
LaVergne TN
LVHW020427070526
838199LV00004B/311